The Arthritis Helpbook

The Arthritis Helpbook

A Tested Self-Management Program for
Coping with Arthritis and Fibromyalgia

Kate Lorig, R.N., Dr. PH
Professor of Medicine
Director, Patient Education Research Center
Stanford University School of Medicine

James F. Fries, M.D.
Professor of Medicine
Stanford University School of Medicine

CONTRIBUTORS
Maureen R. Gecht-Silver, OTR/L, MPH,
    Clinical Instructor in Family Medicine, UIC
Marian Minor, R.P.T., Ph.D.,
    Professor, University of Missouri
Diana D. Laurent, MPH, Health Educator
Virginia M. González, MPH, Health Educator

Da Capo
LIFE
LONG

A Member of the Perseus Books Group

Copyright © 2006 by Kate R. Lorig and James F. Fries

Adapted from *The Arthritis Helpbook,* Sixth Edition, by Kate R. Lorig, R.N., Dr.P.H. and James F. Fries, M.D.

Text design and production by Eclipse Publishing Services Illustrations in chapters 10 and 11 by Meryl Henderson

Cataloging-in-Publication data for this book is available from the Library of Congress.

First Da Capo Press edition 2006
ISBN-10: 0-7382-1070-6
ISBN-13: 978-0-7382-1070-4

Published by Da Capo Press
A Member of the Perseus Books Group
www.dacapopress.com

Da Capo Press books are available at special discounts for bulk purchases in the U.S. by corporations, institutions, and other organizations. For more information, please contact the Special Markets Department at the Perseus Books Group, 11 Cambridge Center, Cambridge, MA 02142, or call (800) 255-1514 or (617) 252-5298, or email special.markets@perseusbooks.com.

4 5 6 7 8 9 – 10 09 08

Contents

A Note to Readers

This book is not meant to replace medical care. Rather, it is a supplement to that care. Most doctors do not have the time or take the time to explain exercises or pain-management techniques to you in enough detail to help you very much. Therefore, we hope this book will assist both you and your physician. All of the advice and activities that we describe have been reviewed by many, many doctors, physical therapists, occupational therapists, nutritionists, and nurses, including the entire staff of the Stanford Arthritis Center. They represent a sound program essentially the same as that recommended by most health authorities today. If you have particular questions please talk them over with your doctor.

We would like you to feel that you are part of our cast of thousands. If you have comments or suggestions please send them to us by writing:

Stanford Patient Education Research Center
1000 Welch Road, Suite 204
Palo Alto, CA 94304
U.S.A.
self-management@stanford.edu

Your suggestions will be reviewed and considered for our next edition.

To all of you who helped in the past and whom we couldn't name, many thanks, and to those of you who are just joining, a hearty welcome.

K. L.
J. F. F.
Stanford, California
January 2006

Part I

Understanding Those Aches and Pains

Chapter 1
Arthritis: What Is It?

Arthritis. Fibromyalgia. The very words evoke a specter of fear and pain. People think of getting old, being unable to get around, and of becoming more dependent upon others. The terms carry with them a sense of hopelessness and futility. But the very opposite should be true. All arthritis and fibromyalgia can be helped.

In order to understand how to work with your condition, it is necessary to know a little about it. In fact, arthritis is not just a single disease. There are over 120 kinds of arthritis, all of which have something to do with one or more joints in the body. Even the word *arthritis* is misleading. The *arth-* part comes from the Greek word meaning "joint," while *-itis* means "inflammation or infection." Thus, the word *arthritis* means "inflammation of the joint." The problem is that, in many kinds of arthritis, the joint is not inflamed. A better definition might be "problems with the joint, or the ligaments, tendons, and muscles near the joint." "Rheumatism" is a broader term that encompasses all kinds of pain and stiffness in the muscles and joints.

Now that you understand what *arthritis* means, the next step is to understand what a joint looks like and what the various parts do.

A joint is a meeting of two bones for the purpose of allowing movement. It has the following six parts.

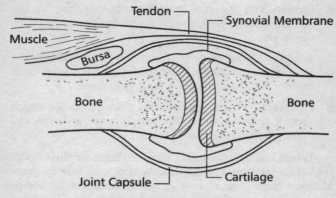

Where arthritis attacks.

1. **Cartilage.** The end of each bone is covered with cartilage, a tough material that cushions and protects the ends of the bone. To get some idea of what cartilage is like, feel the middle of your nose or your ears. These are also made of cartilage. Cartilage in meat is gristle.

2. **Synovial membrane (synovial sac).** Around each joint is the synovial sac, which protects the joint and also secretes the synovial fluid, which oils the joint. In fact, this fluid has many times the lubricating power of oil. Synovial fluid is a little like egg white.

3. **Bursa.** A bursa is a small sac that is not part of the joint but is near the joint. It contains a fluid that lubricates the movement of muscles: muscle across muscle and muscle across bones. In some ways, it is similar to the synovial sac.

4. **Muscle.** The muscles are elastic tissues that, by becoming shorter and longer, move the bones and thus move you.

5. **Tendon.** The tendons are fibrous cords that attach the muscles to the bones. You can feel them on the back of your hand or in the back of your knee.

6. **Ligament.** The ligaments are fibrous cords, much shorter than tendons, that attach bone to bone and make up the joint capsules.

When someone says, "I have arthritis or fibromyalgia," it means that something is wrong with one or more of these parts. For example, when the synovial membrane becomes inflamed, this is true arthritis. The joint is inflamed. However, if the muscle becomes stretched from overexercise or is injured, this is not arthritis. The joint itself is not affected.

In each major kind of arthritis, a different joint part is involved. In *rheumatoid arthritis,* the problem is chiefly *synovitis,* an inflammation of the synovial membrane. This inflammation must be reduced with medication in addition to your self-management program. In *ankylosing spondylitis,* the problem is an *enthesopathy,* an inflammation where the ligaments attach to the bone. This inflammation also needs to be suppressed by medication, and the affected joints need to be regularly and vigorously stretched. In *osteoarthritis,* the problem is a breakdown of the joint cartilage, but it can be helped by exercise and proper use of your joints. In *gout,* the problem is crystals in the joint space that cause inflammation and pain. In *fibromyalgia,* the problem is not the joint, but the muscles and ligaments. Each kind of arthritis is different and requires different medical treatment. However, the self-management techniques are very similar for most types of arthritis.

The table on pages 6–7 gives a quick overview of the three most common types of arthritis: rheumatoid arthritis, osteoarthritis, and fibromyalgia.

If you are interested in knowing more about these and other types of arthritis, read *Arthritis: A Take Care of Yourself Health Guide*, by Dr. James F. Fries (Cambridge, Mass.: Da Capo Press, 1999), or contact your local Arthritis Foundation or Arthritis Society for information.

Types of Arthritis

Pathology	Rheumatoid arthritis	Osteoarthritis	Fibromyalgia
What happens	Inflammation of synovial membrane, bone destruction, damage to ligaments, tendons, cartilage, joint capsule.	Cartilage degeneration; bone regeneration (growth) may result in bone spurs.	Unknown. Accompanied by sleep disturbance and prolonged muscle contraction.
Joints affected	Symmetrical: wrists, knees, knuckles (both sides of body).	Hands, spine, knees, hips. May be one-sided.	Joints not affected. Certain tender points. Muscles, ligaments, tendons may be affected.
Features and symptoms	Swelling, redness, warmth, pain, tenderness, nodules, fatigue, stiffness, muscle aches fever.	Localized pain, stiffness; bony knobs of end joints of fingers; usually not much swelling.	Overall aching, morning stiffness, fatigue. Sleep disturbance.
Long-term prognosis	Less aggressive with time; deformity can often be prevented.	Less pain for some, more pain and disability for others; few severely disabled.	Usually improves slowly over time. Pain and fatigue may be disabling in some; most are not disabled.

Types of Arthritis

Pathology	Rheumatoid arthritis	Osteoarthritis	Fibromyalgia
Age at onset	Adults in twenties to fifties, children approaching adolescence.	Forty-five to ninety; most of us have some features with increasing age.	Thirties to fifties.
Sex	75% female.	Males and females equally.	More frequently female.
Heredity	Familial tendency.	The form with knobby fingers can be familial.	Unknown at this time.
Tests	Rheumatoid factor (80%), blood tests, X-rays, examination of joint fluid.	X-rays.	Tender point exam, sometimes blood tests to exclude other conditions (thyroid tests, sedimentation rate).
Treatment	Reduce inflammation. Balanced exercise program, joint protection, weight control, relaxation, heat, sometimes medication and/or surgery.	Maintain activity level. Exercise, joint protection, weight control, relaxation, heat, sometimes medication and/or surgery.	Exercise, heat, relaxation, sometimes medication for pain and/or for enhancing sleep.

Chapter 2

Rheumatoid Arthritis: Inflamed Joints

Rheumatoid arthritis (RA) is more than just arthritis. Indeed, many doctors call it "rheumatoid disease" to emphasize its widespread nature. The name is trying awkwardly to say the same thing; *rheum-* refers to the stiffness, body aching, and fatigue that often accompany rheumatoid arthritis. People with RA often describe feeling much as though they have a virus, with fatigue and aching in the muscles, except that, unlike a usual viral illness, the condition may persist for many years.

About one half of one percent of the population has rheumatoid arthritis, about 20 million people around the world. Most of these people (about three-quarters) are women. The condition usually appears in middle life, in the forties or fifties, although it can begin at any age. Rheumatoid arthritis in children is quite different. Rheumatoid arthritis has been medically identified for about two hundred years, although bone changes in the skeletons of some Mexican Indian groups suggest that the disease may have been around for thousands of years.

Since RA is so common, and because it can sometimes be severe, it is a major international health problem. It can result in difficulties with employment and problems with daily activities and can put a severe stress on family relationships. In its most severe forms, and without good treatment, it can result in deformities of the joints. Fortunately, most people with RA do better than this, and most can lead normal or nearly normal lives. Fear of rheumatoid arthritis, sometimes greatly exaggerated, can be as harmful as the disease itself.

In RA, the synovial membrane lining in the joint becomes inflamed. We don't have a good explanation as to why this inflammation starts, but the cells in the membrane divide and grow, and inflammatory cells come into the joint. Because of the bulk of these inflammatory cells, the joint becomes swollen and feels puffy or boggy to the touch. The increased blood flow that is a feature of the inflammation makes the joint warm. The cells release chemicals (called enzymes) into the joint space and the enzymes cause further irritation and pain. If the process continues for years, the enzymes may gradually digest the cartilage and bone of the joint, actually eating away parts of the bone.

This, then, is rheumatoid arthritis, a process in which inflammation of the joint membrane, over many years, can cause damage to the joint itself.

Features

Swelling and pain in one or more joints, lasting at least six weeks, are required for a diagnosis of rheumatoid arthritis. Usually both sides of the body are affected similarly, and the arthritis is said to be "symmetrical." Often there are slight differences between the two sides, usually the right side being slightly worse in right-handed people and vice versa. Occasionally the condition skips about in an erratic fashion. The wrists and knuckles are almost always involved. The knees and the joints of the ball of the foot are often involved as well, and any joint can be affected. Of the knuckles, those at the base of the fingers are most frequently painful, while the joints at the ends of the fingers are often normal.

Lumps, usually between the size of a pea and a moth-ball, may form beneath the skin. These *rheumatoid nodules* are most commonly located near the elbow at the place where you rest your arms on the table, but they can pop up anywhere. Each represents an inflammation of a small blood vessel. Nodules come and go during the course of the illness and usually are not a big problem. They tend to occur in people with the most severe kinds of RA. In rare cases, they become sore or infected, particularly if they are located around the ankle. Even more rarely, they form in the lungs or elsewhere inside the body.

Laboratory tests can sometimes help a doctor recognize rheumatoid arthritis. The *rheumatoid factor* or *latex fixation* is the most commonly used blood test. Although this test may be negative in the first several months, it is eventually positive in about 80% of people with RA. The rheumatoid factor is actually an antibody to certain body proteins and can sometimes be found in individuals with other diseases. Some doctors think that it is a way the body fights the disease; others think that it may play a role in causing the joint damage.

The *sed rate* is another frequently used blood test. This test's full name is *erythrocyte sedimentation rate;* the name sometimes is abbreviated ESR. The test doesn't help in diagnosis, but it does help tell the severity of the disease. A high sed rate (over 30 or so) suggests that the disease is quite active. The C-Reactive Protein (CRP) test also measures the amount of inflammation. The joint fluid is sometimes examined in rheumatoid arthritis in order to look at the inflammatory cells or to make sure that the joint is not infected with bacteria.

X-rays are not very helpful in the initial diagnosis of rheumatoid arthritis. It is unusual for changes to be seen in the bones or cartilage in the first few months of the disease, even when it is most severe. X-rays can help the doctor determine if damage to the bones or cartilage has occurred as the disease progresses. Some doctors like to get baseline X-rays to compare with later X-rays. Simple hand X-rays probably should be done in the first year of disease and every two or three years thereafter.

Most people with RA notice problems in parts of their bodies other than the joints themselves. Usually there are general problems such as muscle aches, fatigue, muscle stiffness (particularly in the morning), and even a low fever. Morning stiffness is often considered a hallmark of RA and is sometimes termed the *gel phenomenon*. After a rest period or even after just sitting motionless for a few minutes, the whole body feels stiff and is difficult to move. After a period of loosening up, motion becomes easier and less painful. People often have problems with fluid accumulation, particularly around the ankles. Rarely, the rheumatoid disease may attack other body tissues, including the whites of the eyes, the nerves, the small arteries, and the lungs. Anemia (low red-blood-cell count) is quite common, although it is seldom severe enough to need any treatment. Some patients will develop *Sjögren's,* or sicca syndrome, in which the tear fluids and the saliva dry up, causing dry eyes and dry mouth. This happens because the lacrimal (tear) glands and the salivary glands become involved in the rheumatoid process.

There can be unusual features that are due to the inflammation of the joint membrane. A *Baker's cyst* can form behind the knees and may feel like a tumor. It is just the synovial sac full of fluid, but it can extend down into the back of the calf and may cause pain. Or the fluid in the joint can become infected and require immediate treatment. Suspect infection if a single joint, usually a knee, becomes suddenly and severely worse.

Rheumatoid arthritis is one of the most complicated and mysterious diseases known. It is a challenge to patient and physician alike. Fortunately, the course of RA can be dramatically changed in most individuals. New treatment strategies are much more effective than the old ones. More so than with any other form of arthritis, RA requires you to develop an effective partnership with your doctor, as discussed in Chapter 17.

Prognosis
(What Will Happen in the Future)

Rheumatoid arthritis is the condition that most people think of when they hear the word *arthritis*. An image that comes to mind is of a person in a wheelchair, with swollen knees and twisted hands. True, many such people have rheumatoid arthritis. On balance, rheumatoid arthritis is the most destructive kind of arthritis known. Erosion of the bone itself, rupture of tendons, and slippage of the joints can result in crippling. But most people with rheumatoid arthritis do very much better than this. Many of the serious problems can be prevented by good, early treatment.

Often it is hard for persons with RA and their relatives to appreciate that inflammation in even the worst forms of rheumatoid arthritis tends to lessen with time. The arthritis usually becomes less aggressive. The inflammation (synovitis) is less active and the fatigue and stiffness decrease. New joints are less likely to become involved after several years of disease. But even though the disease becomes less violent, any destruction of bones and ligaments that occurred in earlier years will persist. Thus, deformities usually will not improve, even though no new damage is occurring. Hence, it is important to treat the disease correctly in the early years so that the joints will work well after the disease inflammation subsides.

Treatment

Treatment programs for RA are often complicated and can be confusing. In this section we give the broad outlines for sound management. But you need to work out with your doctor the combination of measures that is best for you. It has been said that the person who has himself for a doctor has a fool for a patient. In many areas of medicine, and for some kinds of arthritis, this is not true; you can do just as well looking out for yourself. But with rheumatoid arthritis, you do need a doctor. Indeed, with rheumatoid arthritis, we strongly believe that you should be seen early in the course of the disease by a specialist in arthritis, a rheumatologist. In this way, the critical early treatment can begin at the right time. Only rheumatologists are familiar with the latest and most effective RA treatments.

First, some common sense. Your RA may be with you, on and off, for months or years. The best treatments are those that will help you maintain a life that is as nearly normal as possible. Often the worst treatments are those that offer immediate relief. They may allow joint damage to progress or may cause delayed side effects that ultimately make you feel worse. So you must develop some patience with the disease and with its management. You have to adjust your thinking to operate in the same slow time scale that the disease uses. You and your doctor will want to anticipate problems before they occur so that they may be avoided. The adjustment to a long-term illness, with the necessity to plan treatment programs that may take months to get results, is a difficult psychological task. This adjustment will be one of your hardest jobs in battling your arthritis.

Synovitis is the underlying problem. The inflammation of the joint membrane releases enzymes that very slowly damage the joint structures. Good treatment reduces this inflammation and stops the damage.

Painkillers can increase comfort but do not decrease the arthritis. In fact, pain per se helps to protect the joints by discouraging too much use. Therefore, in RA it is important to treat pain by treating the inflammation that causes the pain. By and large, pain relievers such as codeine, Percodan, Darvon, or Demerol must be avoided. (To learn more, read Chapter 20.)

The proper balance between rest and exercise is hard to understand. Rest reduces the inflammation, and this is good. But rest also lets joints get stiff and muscles get weak. With too much rest, tendons become weaker and bones get softer. Obviously, this is bad. So moderation is the basic principle. It may help you to know that your body usually gives you the right signals about what to do and what not to do. If it hurts too much, don't do it. If you don't seem to have much problem with an activity, go ahead. As a rule, if you continue to have pain caused by exercise for more than two hours after exercising, you have done too much.

A particularly painful joint may require a splint to help it rest. Still, you will want to exercise the joint by stretching it gently in different directions to keep it from getting stiff. You will not want to use a splint for too long, or you may want to use it just at night. As the joint gets better, you will want to begin using the joint, gently at first, but slowly progressing to more and more activity. In general, favor activities that build good muscle tone, not those that build great muscle strength. Walking and swimming are better than moving furniture and lifting heavy weights, since tasks requiring a lot of strength put a lot of stress across the joint. And regular exercises done daily are better than occasional sprees of activity that stress joints that are not ready for so much exertion.

Common sense and a regular, long-term program are the keys to success. Should you take a nap after lunch? Yes, if you're tired. Should you undertake some particular outing? Go on a trip? You know your regular daily activity level. Common sense will help you answer most such questions. Full normal activity should be approached gradually, with a long-term conditioning program that includes rest when needed and gradual increases in activity during nonresting periods.

Physical therapists and occupational therapists can often help with specific advice and helpful hints. The best therapists will help you develop your own program for home exercise and will teach you the exercises and activities that will help your joints. However, don't expect the therapist to do your program for you. Your rest and exercise program cannot consist solely of formal sessions at a rehabilitation facility. You must take the responsibility to build the habits that will, on a daily basis, protect and strengthen your joints. It is important to start exercise and proper use of your joints before you have problems. These are good preventive measures.

Medications are required by almost all patients with rheumatoid arthritis, and often must be continued for years. Great progress has been made recently with disease-modifying antirheumatic drugs (DMARDs), causing a virtual revolution in the treatment of rheumatoid arthritis (see Chapter 19). These crucial drugs should be prescribed early in the course of the disease. The most important rule now is "Don't do too little, too late." At present, the DMARD drugs are Plaquenil, Azulfidine, gold shots, oral gold (Ridaura), penicillamine, methotrexate, Imuran, leflunomide, minocycline, cyclosporin, and the cytokine treatments. More are under development. The great majority of patients with RA should be taking a DMARD or a combination of DMARDs at all times.

Less powerful anti-inflammatory drugs are similar to aspirin. Aspirin is a valuable drug when used as detailed in Chapter 18. Every patient with RA should become familiar with the uses of aspirin, which, used correctly, can be a good analgesic drug with an acceptable level of side effects. Aspirin variants, such as Disalcid and Trilisate, may better protect the stomach lining. Drugs roughly similar to aspirin are called *nonsteroidal anti-inflammatory drugs* (NSAIDs) and are also frequently used. Examples of such drugs are Lodine, Relafen, Motrin, Voltaren, Naprosyn, Indocin, and Feldene. The new COX-2 selective inhibitors are among the least toxic drugs on the stomach but may pose risks to the heart. There is increasing use of acetaminophen (Tylenol), which is not an anti-inflammatory drug but helps with pain and is quite safe. For more information on these drugs, see Chapter 18.

Drugs such as sulfasalazine (Azulfidine), auranofin (Ridaura), or hydroxychloroquine (Plaquenil) (page 298) are often used as the first DMARDs. Gold injections (page 295) are often very helpful and sometimes result in complete disappearance of the arthritis if used early enough. Methotrexate has become the most frequently used, and probably the best, DMARD. Penicillamine can also result in dramatic improvement. Azathioprine (Imuran), leflunomide (Arava), minocycline, and the cytokine treatments are also in this category.

Corticosteroids, most frequently prednisone, are strong hormones with formidable long-term side effects. Their use is controversial in rheumatoid arthritis; some physicians feel that they should almost never be used, while others use them only in very small doses, except in unusual circumstances.

See chapters 18, 19, and 20 for detailed discussions of individual drugs.

Surgery sometimes can restore the function of a damaged joint. Hip replacement, knee replacement, shoulder replacement, synovectomy of the knee, metatarsal head resection, and synovectomy of the knuckles are among the most frequent operations. These are discussed in Chapter 21.

Chapter 3

Osteoarthritis: Worn Cartilage

Osteoarthritis (OA), also known as osteoarthrosis or degenerative joint disease (DJD), is the kind of arthritis that almost everybody gets. It is increasingly common with age, and, because of its relationship to the aging process, it is not as responsive to medical treatment as we might like. However, there are many things you can do for yourself to alleviate this disease. Fortunately, osteoarthritis is usually a much less severe form of arthritis than rheumatoid arthritis. The changes in the skeleton that occur with age are inevitable, and they cause symptoms in many people but severe symptoms in very few.

Osteoarthritis used to be thought of as the inevitable result of "wear and tear." In fact, most activities with a lot of "wear" don't seem to cause much "tear," and authorities now recognize the need for exercise to strengthen the joints, both before and after signs of arthritis have developed. Exercise will very seldom harm someone with OA. On the other hand, being inactive can cause a great deal of harm.

The tissue involved in osteoarthritis is the cartilage. This gristle material faces the ends of the bones and forms the surface of the joint on both sides. Our ears and nose are also made of cartilage. Gristle is tough, somewhat elastic, and very durable. The cartilage, or gristle, does not have a blood supply, so it gets its oxygen and nutrition from the surrounding joint fluid. In this it is aided by being elastic and able to absorb fluid. When we use a joint, the pressure squeezes fluid and waste products out of the cartilage, and when the pressure is relieved, the fluid seeps back, together with oxygen and nutrients. Hence, the health of the cartilage depends on use of the joint. Over many years, the cartilage may become frayed and may even wear away entirely. When this happens, the bone surface on one side of the joint grates against the bone on the other side of the joint, providing a much less elastic joint surface. With time, the opposing bony surfaces may become polished, a process called *eburnation*. As this happens, the joint may again move more smoothly and cause less discomfort. This is one of the reasons it is important to continue to use painful joints.

The difference between the terms *osteoarthritis* and *osteoarthrosis* has to do with the question of inflammation. The suffix *-itis* denotes inflammation, and with osteoarthritis very little inflammation is to be found. Hence, some experts prefer the term osteoarthrosis, which does not imply inflammation. Otherwise, both words mean the same.

There are three common types of osteoarthritis. The first and mildest causes knobby enlargement of the finger joints. The end joints of the fingers become bony and the hands begin to assume the appearance we associate with old age. The other joints of the fingers may also be involved. This kind of arthritis (or arthrosis) usually causes little difficulty beyond the cosmetic. There may be some stiffness, and there can be some pain, particularly when the bony knobs are growing.

The second form of osteoarthritis involves the spine and is sometimes called *degenerative joint disease*. Bony growths (spurs) appear on the spine in the neck region or in the lower back. Usually the bony growths are associated with some narrowing of the space between the vertebrae. This time the disk, rather than cartilage, is the material that becomes frayed. Changes in the spine begin early in life in almost all of us but cause long-term symptoms relatively seldom.

The third form of osteoarthritis involves the weight-bearing joints, almost always the hips or the knees. These problems can be quite severe.

It is possible to have all three kinds of osteoarthritis or any two of them, but often a person will have only one.

Individuals who have had fractures near a joint or have a congenital malformation at a joint seem to develop osteoarthritis in those joints at an earlier age. But, as noted, the usual description of this arthritis as "wear and tear" is not accurate. While excessive wear and tear on the joint can theoretically result in damage, activity helps the joint remain supple and lubricated, and this tends to cancel out the theoretically bad effects.

Careful studies of people who regularly put a lot of stress on joints (such as individuals who operate pneumatic drills or run long distances on hard paved surfaces) have been unable to show a relationship between these activities and the development of arthritis. Hence, intensive activity does not predispose you to arthritis any more than intensive activity predisposes you to heart disease. In fact, the very opposite may be true. On the other hand, injury to the joint, as in knee injuries in football players, may lead to osteoarthritis in the injured joint. Excess body weight can lead to OA of the hip or knee.

Features

The bony knobs that form around the end joints of the fingers are called *Heberden's nodes,* after the British doctor who first described them. Similar knobs can be found in the middle joints of the fingers. Usually, the bony enlargement occurs slowly over a period of years and is not even noticed. In most cases, all of the fingers are involved more or less equally.

There is an interesting variation of osteoarthritis in which the bony swelling occurs over only three or four weeks in a single finger joint. The sudden swelling causes redness and soreness until the process is complete; then it stops hurting altogether. This syndrome is seen in women in their forties, earlier than the more usual form of osteoarthritis. These patients frequently have other family members with the same problem. This "familial" form of osteoarthrosis doesn't really seem very much worse over the long run, but one joint after another may suddenly develop a bony knob over a short period.

Osteoarthritis of the spine does not cause symptoms unless there is pressure on one of the nerves or irritation of some of the other structures of the back. If a doctor tells you that you have arthritis in your spine, do not assume that any pain you feel is necessarily related to that arthritis. Most people with X-rays showing arthritis of the spine do not have any problem at all from the bone spurs seen on the X-ray; the pain is from some nearby structure such as a ligament or muscle.

Osteoarthritis of the weight-bearing joints, particularly the hip and knee, develops slowly and often involves both sides of the body. Pain in the joint may remain fairly constant or may wax and wane over a period of years. In severe cases, walking may be difficult or even impossible. Fluid may accumulate in the affected joint, giving it a swollen appearance, or a knee may wobble a bit when weight is placed on it. In the knee, the osteoarthritis usually affects the inner or the outer half of the joint more than the other; this may result in the leg becoming bowed or splayed and may cause difficulty walking.

X-rays can be helpful in evaluating osteoarthritis. The two major findings on the X-ray are narrowing of the joint space and the presence of bony spurs, or *osteophytes*. X-rays pass right through cartilage. Hence, in a normal joint the X-ray looks as though the two bones are separated by a space; in reality, the apparent space is filled with cartilage. As the cartilage is frayed, the apparent joint space on the X-ray narrows until the two bones may touch each other. Spurs are little bone growths that appear alongside the places where the cartilage has degenerated. The bony growth provides a larger joint surface. It is as though the body is trying to react to a cartilage problem by providing more surface area for the joint, so as to distribute the weight more evenly. In addition, X-rays can sometimes show the holes through which the nerves pass and can indicate whether these holes are narrowed.

Blood tests are not very helpful in diagnosing osteoarthritis. There is nothing wrong with the rest of the body, so all the tests are normal.

Prognosis (What Will Happen in the Future)

Prognosis is good for all forms of osteoarthritis. When you think of an aging process, you tend to think of a progressive condition that will continue to get worse and worse. That is not necessarily the case. Osteoarthritis may get worse for a while and then become stable for a long time. A joint that has lost its cartilage may not function well at first, but with use the bone may be molded and polished so that a smooth and more functional joint is developed. Even in the worst cases, osteoarthritis progresses slowly. You have lots of time to think about what kinds of treatment are likely to help. If a surgical decision is needed, you can consider for some time whether you want an operation or not. Crippling from osteoarthritis is relatively rare, and most people with osteoarthritis can remain essentially free of symptoms.

Treatment

The revolution in treatment of OA is to emphasize the role of exercise. The consequence of osteoarthritis can be loss of physical function. Because of pain, you tend to be less active, and this accelerates the loss of function. People used to be told to "take it easy." Now it is recognized that even the first symptoms of osteoarthritis are a signal for a regular, dedicated exercise program to increase heart, muscle, ligament, tendon, and bone strength.

Joints should be exercised through their full range of motion several times a day. If weight-bearing joints are involved, body weight should be kept under control; obesity accelerates the rate of damage. The most helpful exercises seem to be swimming, walking, and bicycling, which are easy, can be gradually increased, and are smooth rather than jerky. Strengthening exercises, described in Chapter 11, can also be of help. Exercise should be regular. Thus, if you start getting some osteoarthritis, it is not a signal to begin to tone down your life, but rather to develop a sensible regular exercise program to strengthen the bones and ligaments surrounding the affected joints and to preserve mobility in joints that are developing spurs. (For details on flexibility exercises, see Chapter 10.)

Drug therapy is used to control discomfort. Aspirin in moderate doses is frequently helpful. Acetaminophen (Tylenol), which is the safest analgesic drug, has been found to be just as good for many people as the more toxic (and usually more expensive) alternatives.

Ibuprofen and other anti-inflammatory drugs (NSAIDs) may be helpful for some people, and these are discussed in Chapter 18. We try to avoid codeine or other strong pain relievers because pain is a signal to the body that helps protect a diseased joint; it is important that this signal be received. (For details on pain management, see Chapter 14.) Glucosamine and chondroitin sulfate are not scientifically proven to be useful, but some patients report less pain after taking these agents.

Frequently, some kinds of devices can assist. A cane may be helpful; less commonly, crutches are needed. Occasionally, special shoes or lifts on one side of the foot may be helpful.

Most physicians now believe that symptomatic osteoarthritis may be substantially prevented by good health habits. If you are active, maintain a lean body weight, exercise your muscles and joints regularly to nourish cartilage, and let your common sense tell you when you have done too much and something hurts, your joints should last a lifetime. Like exercise of the heart muscle, exercise of the muscles and joints provides reserve for the occasional strenuous activities we all encounter. Exercise builds strong tissues that last a long time.

Injection of osteoarthritic joints with corticosteroids is occasionally helpful, and sometimes removal of some fluid from a joint may help. Usually, however, injections do not help much since there is not much inflammation to be suppressed. Injections should not be frequently repeated, because the injection itself may damage the cartilage and the bone. Injection with lubricating substances, such as Hylan (Synvisc), may give some relief for some people but it is not frequently needed.

Surgery can be dramatically effective for people with severe osteoarthritis of the weight-bearing joints. Total hip replacement is the most important operation yet devised for any form of arthritis. Practically all individuals are free of pain after the surgery, and many walk normally and carry out normal activities. Total knee replacement is a more recent operation and gives far better results than the knee surgery available just a few years ago. Surgery is never urgent, and you and your doctor will want to decide when the discomfort or the limitation of your walking has become bad enough to warrant the discomfort, costs, and small risk associated with the operation. (For more information on surgery, see Chapter 21.)

Chapter 4

Osteoporosis: Brittle Bones

Osteoporosis is a bone disease in which the bones lose calcium, become more brittle, and break more easily. While anyone can have osteoporosis, it is most common in elderly people, particularly women. Because of osteoporosis, one in five women breaks a hip before the age of seventy-five. Fractures of the spine, resulting in pain, decrease in height, and a forward deformity of the spine (Dowager's Hump) are even more common. Inactivity makes osteoporosis worse.

Although the best protection from osteoporosis is prevention, thankfully, we now have some effective treatments. As with all kinds of arthritis and rheumatism, consistent good health practices are crucial. This starts with a lifestyle that excludes smoking and drinking too much alcohol.

The following pages outline the healthy habits that are useful in preventing and dealing with osteoporosis.

Dietary Calcium

Our bones cannot maintain their strength unless our bodies regularly receive an adequate supply of calcium. Recently, the National Institutes of Health (NIH) Consensus Development Conference on optimal calcium intake concluded that millions of Americans are not getting nearly enough calcium in their diets and that the

Recommended Calcium Intake

Group	Recommended Intake (in milligrams of calcium)
INFANTS	
Birth to 6 months	210
6 months to 1 year	270
CHILDREN	
1 to 3 years	500
4 to 8 years	800
MALES	
9 to 18	1,300
19 to 50	1,000
Over 50	1,200
FEMALES	
9 to 18	1,300
19 to 50	1,000
Over 50	1,200

official recommended daily allowance (RDA) for calcium may not be adequate for some age groups. The table above shows the recommended amounts of calcium for different ages.

To bring your calcium intake up to 1,000 mg, eat two or three servings of milk products a day (nonfat milk is best) and regularly include other calcium-rich foods in your meals. Also, moderate the amount of salt and meat you eat. (Chapter 13 discusses how to do this.) Excessive amounts of sodium or meat can increase your need for calcium.

The table "Food Sources of Calcium" on pages 28–29 gives you a good idea of the types of food that are relatively rich in calcium. Notice that you can get significant quantities of calcium without drinking milk. Yogurts, cheeses, and hot cereals made with milk all supply calcium. Canned salmon, mackerel, and sardines are excellent sources of calcium *if* you eat the soft bones.

Supplemental Calcium

It is better to get calcium from your foods than to rely on calcium supplements. But if you cannot eat two or more servings of dairy products every day, or if you want to take in more than 1,000 mg of calcium, supplements can provide practical help.

In general, choose a supplement that contains between 500 and 1,000 mg (50 to 100% of the RDA) of "elemental calcium." "Elemental calcium" means the actual amount of calcium in the pill. Take one or two full doses a day, depending on your needs, not more.

As the "Supplemental Calcium" table on page 30 illustrates, the elemental calcium in a supplement can come from any of several different calcium compounds. Less expensive store-brand supplements are usually fine; use the product that suits you best. Sometimes inexpensive calcium tablets won't dissolve in your stomach, however, so try this test. Put a tablet in half a glass of water for thirty minutes. It should become shaggy and partly dissolve. If not, fill the glass the rest of the way with vinegar, stir gently, and wait another half hour. If the tablet is still not dissolved, it is not a good product for you.

Myths About Calcium

1. "Calcium causes bone spurs." Maintaining a calcium intake of 800 to 1,500 mg a day (or even much higher) will not cause bone spurs.

Food Sources of Calcium

Food	Amount	Calcium (approx.)
LOW-FAT AND NONFAT MILK PRODUCTS		
Nonfat milk	1 cup (235 ml)	300 mg
Low-fat milk (1% fat)	1 cup (235 ml)	300 mg
Low-fat milk (2% fat)	1 cup (235 ml)	295 mg
Nonfat dry milk powder	3 tbsp (45 ml)	280 mg
Nonfat yogurt (plain)	1 cup (235 ml)	450 mg
Low-fat yogurt (plain)	1 cup (235 ml)	415 mg
Low-fat cottage cheese (2% fat)	1 cup (235 ml)	155 mg
Part-skim ricotta cheese	1/2 cup (120 ml)	335 mg
Part-skim mozzarella	2 oz (56 g)	365 mg
FULL-FAT MILK PRODUCTS		
Whole milk (3.5% fat)	1 cup (235 ml)	290 mg
Whole-milk yogurt (plain)	1 cup (235 ml)	275 mg
Swiss cheese	1 oz (28 g)	270 mg
Cheddar cheese	1 oz (28 g)	205 mg
Processed American cheese	1 oz (28 g)	125 mg

Food Sources of Calcium

Food	Amount	Calcium (approx.)
FULL-FAT MILK PRODUCTS *(continued)*		
Frozen yogurt	1 cup (235 ml)	175 mg
Ice cream (regular, 10% fat)	1 cup (235 ml)	175 mg
Ice cream (rich, 16% fat)	1 cup (235 ml)	150 mg
OTHER CALCIUM-RICH FOODS		
Almonds	1 oz (28 g)	75 mg
Broccoli (boiled)	1 cup (235 ml)	180 mg
Corn tortilla	1	40 mg
Great northern beans (boiled)	1 cup (235 ml)	120 mg
Kale (boiled)	1 cup (235 ml)	95 mg
Navy beans (boiled)	1 cup (235 ml)	130 mg
Pinto beans (boiled)	1 cup (235 ml)	80 mg
Tofu (soybean curd)	1/2 cup (120 ml)	130 mg
Canned salmon (including bones)	3 oz (84 g)	190 mg
Canned sardines (including bones)	1 oz (28 g)	85 mg

For most people, low-fat and nonfat dairy products are better choices than full-fat products. See Chapter 13.

Supplemental Calcium

Sources of Supplemental Calcium	Elemental Calcium Content
Calcium carbonate (in oyster-shell calcium, BioCal, Caltrate 600, OsCal, Tums)	40%
Calcium citrate (in CitraCal)	21%
Calcium lactate (available in store-brand products)	13%

2. "Calcium causes kidney stones." While it is prudent to avoid calcium intakes that exceed 2,000 to 2,500 mg a day, consuming a total of 800 to 1,500 mg a day is unlikely to lead to kidney stones. If you have had kidney stones in the past, you should check with your doctor before starting a calcium supplement. Otherwise, just be sure to drink plenty of fluids whenever you take a calcium tablet.

3. "Calcium causes constipation." Large doses of calcium can cause constipation in some people. But the problem generally can be avoided by drinking plenty of fluids and eating foods high in fiber. See Chapter 16 for more information.

Hormones

Calcium by itself will not stop bone loss. The body needs a stimulus to absorb the calcium and to get it into the bone. The best stimuli are estrogen therapy for post-menopausal women and adequate weight-bearing exercise for everybody. The use of hormones such as estrogen after menopause has long been a topic of controversy. This is a subject every woman should discuss with her physician. The following discussion is to help you understand some of the issues.

Estrogen

There are two female hormones, estrogen and progestin. These hormones are normally created during the menstrual cycle. After menopause, their levels fall greatly. Taking supplemental estrogen after menopause seems to protect against osteoporosis. However, estrogen is believed by some to increase the likelihood of endometrial cancer (cancer of the lining of the uterus). When progestin is taken with the estrogen, a number of health problems may result, including cancer, stroke, and heart disease. These hormones also help prevent hot flashes, vaginal dryness, and skin wrinkling. The decision to take no hormone, one hormone (estrogen), or a combination of the two is a personal one and should be discussed with a physician. Most physicians have become more cautious in routinely recommending estrogen for postmenopausal women.

Other Treatments

Calcitonin

An approved alternative to estrogen-replacement therapy for treatment of osteoporosis is salmon calcitonin. Calcitonin can actually help build back strong bones, not just slow down the process of bone loss. The major drawback to the treatment has been its expense and the need for patients to learn how to self-administer injections. The medication may cause transient flushing and nausea in about 20% of patients. Calcitonin administration by nasal spray is now possible and is considerably easier.

Biphosphonates

Etidronate (Didronel) was the first of a class of drugs called biphosphonates, followed by Clordronate. These "first-generation" biphosphonates were usually given for a two-week period each three months (cyclic therapy), since they don't work if given continuously. These drugs have been shown to produce a small increase in bone density and to decrease the frequency of spine fractures. Because biphosphonates are poorly absorbed, they must be taken on an empty stomach and only with water.

"Second-generation" biphosphonates are now available, led by alendronate (Fosamax) and including pamidronate, tiludronate, and ibandronate. These can be taken continuously and decrease the risk of spinal fractures by 50 to 90%, even in people who have already had a fracture. These drugs can irritate the esophagus, so they are best taken in the morning with a glass of warm water. The standard approach has changed from 10 mg fosomax daily to 10 mg once a week; this is equally effective and better tolerated. The "third-generation" drug residronate appears to cause less stomach irritation.

Vitamin D

Vitamin D comes with sunlight and diet. If you are usually indoors or malnourished, supplementation (as with a multivitamin) may be a good idea.

Fluoride

Slow-release fluoride (25 mg twice a day for twelve months followed by two months off) has been shown to increase bone mass and decrease vertebral fractures but is not yet available in the United States.

Experimental Treatments

Parathyroid fragments and growth factors are under study and appear promising.

Exercise

Weight-bearing exercise is very, very important in maintaining strong bones. The body reacts to such exercise by increasing the calcium content and thus the strength of the bones. Walking is the best example. If at all possible, walk half a mile to a mile (1 to 1.5 km) a day. If this is unrealistic for you, remember that even a little weight-bearing exercise is important. Do as much as you can. For suggestions on developing a walking program, see chapters 9 and 12. Recent research has shown that women need to walk four miles (6 km) a week to get maximal exercise benefit for osteoporosis prevention. This includes all the walking we do in our daily lives. (Note: Swimming is not a weight-bearing exercise.)

Preventing Falls

Unfortunately, it is not always possible to prevent osteoporosis or undo damage already done. Remember, osteoporosis by itself does not cause pain. The pain comes from fractures in the spine or other bones. Thus, avoiding falls is very important to prevent broken bones. The following are a few hints:

▼ Avoid area rugs; they are slippery and have a bad habit of tripping the unwary.

▼ Be sure all stairs have a secure railing that is easy to grasp.

▼ If advised to do so by a health professional, use a cane, stick, or walker. These can be real bone savers.

▼ Even if you don't usually use a cane, consider using one for getting up at night. This is a time when most of us may easily lose our balance and a cane can help prevent bad spills.

▼ Watch for uneven walks, curbs, floors, and so on.

▼ Move the phone to a convenient place so you won't trip over the cord.

▼ Wear shoes that give good support.

▼ Use step stools that are stable and in good repair.

▼ Use nonskid mats in the bathtub and shower and on the bathroom floor. Permanently install grab bars to the wall or the edge of the tub.

▼ If you are unsteady on your feet, sit on a stool with nonskid feet when showering or bathing.

▼ Have light switches at the top and bottom of all stairs.

▼ Be careful not to hold your breath when you are on the toilet. This can cause you to pass out and fall.

Summary:
Preventing and Treating Osteoporosis

There are five things you can do to help prevent and treat osteoporosis:

1. Make positive lifestyle changes: Stop smoking and reduce alcohol consumption.

2. Do some weight-bearing exercises every day.

3. Take adequate calcium by modifying your diet or using a combination of diet and supplements.

4. If advised by your physician, take estrogen, biphosphonates, vitamin D, or sodium fluoride.

5. Make your home and other surroundings fall-safe.

Chapter 5

Fibromyalgia:
Chronic Pain and Fatigue

Fibromyalgia is a common and increasingly recognized condition. In 1990 it was defined in terms of two distinguishing characteristics:

▼ Pain and aching in many parts of the body lasting for at least three months

▼ Local tenderness in eleven of eighteen specified places on the body

Features

The fibromyalgia syndrome (FMS) is a very common condition, affecting perhaps 5 million people in the United States alone and accounting for one out of every six visits to rheumatologists. Patients are more likely to be women, but children, the elderly, and men can also be affected. Their average age is about fifty-five. People with this syndrome also may experience sleep disturbances, severe fatigue, morning stiffness, irritable bowel syndrome, anxiety, and other symptoms, such as trouble remembering things.

The *tender points* are particular body locations that are normally somewhat tender; many readers will be able to identify these points on their own bodies. Firm pressure applied to these areas will hurt anyone, but the person with fibromyalgia experiences great pain when these areas are pressed lightly. For example, about halfway between the neck and the shoulder, one can feel the upper border of the trapezius muscle; at the midpoint of this muscle there is a tender site. Another is the "tennis elbow" site, just about an inch (2.5 cm) down the forearm from the outer bump on the side of the elbow when the palm is turned up; this tender spot may feel like a cord. There are also tender points at the second costochondral junction, on either side of the breastbone and about an inch or two (2.5 to 5 cm) below the collarbone. A fourth site is in the fat pad on the inside portion of the knee. Others are between the shoulder blades and at the base of the skull. A person with fibromyalgia usually has tenderness at most of these places and may have more general tenderness as well.

Half or more of those with fibromyalgia have chronic fatigue. Fatigue may be severe and interfere with activities. Some of the factors that contribute to fatigue are pain, sleep problems, and stress factors. A frequent but not quite universal characteristic of fibromyalgia is sleep disturbance. There is an interruption of slow-wave brain activity, the kind of sleep most restful to the muscles, in many patients. Patients frequently report that upon awakening in the morning they feel as though they never got to sleep at all.

Although the cause of fibromyalgia is unknown, researchers have several theories about causes or triggers of the disease. There is elevation of a pain peptide (substance P) in the cerebrospinal fluid; it may be that there is a new "thermostat" setting for the pain threshold in fibromyalgia patients. Serotonin in the platelets is lower than normal. Fibromyalgia may be associated with changes in muscle metabolism such as decreased blood flow, causing fatigue and decreased strength. Others believe that the syndrome may be triggered by an infectious agent, such as a virus, in susceptible people. Stress is also a frequently reported cause.

Prognosis
(What Will Happen in the Future)

Medically, fibromyalgia carries a fairly good prognosis for most people. There will usually be no crippling, but the discomfort may last for many years or even for life. The pain can vary over a period of months or years but often never fully goes away. In the United States, most fibromyalgia patients are able to work. About 30% have had to reduce the duration or physical exertion associated with their jobs. About 15% are disabled and receiving Social Security disability payments.

Fibromyalgia symptoms may also be seen in many other disease conditions, such as rheumatoid arthritis, lupus, or Sjögren's, which themselves may disturb sleep. The "secondary" fibromyalgia must not be confused with a flare-up of the other condition, since the treatment is different.

Treatment

Treatment for fibromyalgia is usually frustrating for both the patient and the doctor. Often the patient's close family members are equally frustrated. The root cause of the frustration is the difficulty in getting the symptoms to go away.

The doctor is frustrated for many reasons. There are no objective findings to observe. All the trusted tests are negative. Familiar treatments such as anti-inflammatory medications and analgesics don't work well. The patient is often angry and demanding. When the doctor suggests therapy, the patient often responds that it won't work, even before it has been tried. The doctor may not even believe that the condition fibromyalgia exists and finds it all too easy to conclude that "it's all in your head."

The person with fibromyalgia is even more frustrated than the doctor. The person hurts. The job, the family, and the satisfactions of life are all threatened. Drug after drug fails to help. Exercise seems to cause flare-ups. The doctor doesn't get it. The doctor doesn't listen. The patient has trouble being taken seriously. The doctor thinks "it's all in your head," while the patient desperately wants the problem taken care of.

Fibromyalgia is a real condition. The symptoms are real, chronic, and frustrating; they are *not* "all in your head." Chronic pain does do something to your head also, and frustration and anger do not help. You need a doctor who listens, cares, and communicates. The doctor needs a patient who works persistently at the self-management program. There is no magic, but there is help.

Exercise, slowly increased toward full aerobic cardiovascular conditioning and physical tiredness, is the single most important component of treatment. Start slowly; even a minute or two an hour is helpful if you have been completely inactive. For more help with exercise, see Chapter 9. When a patient is able to walk extensively and to swim, hike, or bicycle regularly, we sometimes have seen gradual resolution of the problem in only a few months. In general, impact exercises such as jogging, tennis, or basketball should be avoided. Stretching exercises are important. Pain often gets somewhat worse with a new exercise program before it gets better. Studies have shown that aerobic exercise improves muscle fitness and reduces muscle pain and tenderness. It may also improve sleep.

Progressive muscle relaxation or some other structured relaxation program may also be helpful (see Chapter 14). Heat and massage may give short-term relief. Pain management programs may be beneficial; the most success has come from psychological interventions that include cognitive behavioral therapy. Check with your local chapter of the Arthritis Foundation or the Arthritis

Society for information about fibromyalgia support groups.

Medications that have been commonly used are often given an hour before bedtime and have included amitriptyline (Elavil), cyclobenzaprine (Flexeril), alprazolam (Xanax), and Soma. While these drugs have anti-depressive properties, they are not given for depression, but to improve sleep quality and to relax muscles. These medications increase deep (stage 4) sleep. Ordinary "sleeping pills" are generally not helpful. Nonsteroidal drugs (NSAIDs) such as ibuprofen or naproxen are often used, with variable success. An increasingly common regimen is Prozac in the morning and Elavil in the evening. Side effects of medications are common but can often be avoided by use of lower doses and by changing the timing of the dose. Some authorities recommend vitamin B_1 and B_6 supplements, and benefit has been reported with a combination of magnesium and malic acid.

Part II

Your Self-Management Plan

Chapter 6

Becoming an
Arthritis Self-Manager

Self-management seems like a simple enough term, yet it needs some explaining. Both at home and in the business world, the managers direct the show. They don't do everything themselves; they work with others, including consultants, to get the job done. What makes them managers is that they are responsible for making the decisions and making sure that these decisions are carried through. As an *arthritis* or *fibromyalgia self-manager,* your job is much the same. You gather information and written materials from friends, family, the Arthritis Foundation, Arthritis Society, or Arthritis Care, and the internet. You hire a consultant or a team of consultants: your physician, physical therapist, pharmacists, and other health professionals. Once they have given you their best advice, it is up to you to follow through.

Arthritis, like diabetes and other chronic diseases, needs to be managed. Cures are usually not possible. However, your quality of life and how you are affected by the disease are very much up to you. By learning self-management skills, you can ease the problems of living with arthritis. Have you noticed that some people with severe physical problems get on very well, while others with lesser problems seem to give up on life? The difference is management style.

Being a good manager means working with others, discussing problems, and, most important, understanding that management is a day-to-day job. This doesn't mean that all your decisions will be correct. Managing arthritis, like managing a family, is a complex undertaking. There are many twists, turns, and midcourse corrections.

The key to success in any undertaking is first learning a set of skills and then practicing them until they have been mastered. This is how you acquire the tools to manage arthritis or fibromyalgia. Children cannot read without first learning to recognize the letters of the alphabet. They then learn the sounds of combinations of letters. Later, they learn the meanings of simple words and phrases. It is only after years of practice and mastery that one is able to read a novel. Think about it. The same is true with almost everything we do, from baking a cake to driving a car to planting a garden. These tasks are all based on learning skills and mastering them. Success in arthritis or fibromyalgia self-management is the same. One needs to learn a set of skills and then to practice them daily until success is achieved.

This book is full of information about tools that can help relieve some of the problems caused by your condition. However, we have learned that knowing the skills is not enough. Most of us need a way of incorporating these skills into our daily lives. Unfortunately, whenever we use a new tool, the first attempts are clumsy and slow and show few results. It is easier to return to our old ways than to continue to try to master new and sometimes difficult skills. One of the best ways to master new skills is through goal setting. In the following pages, we will try to outline some of the principles of goal setting. If you use these principles, the success of an arthritis self-management program is almost assured.

You are your own manager. Like any manager of an organization or household, you must do the following:

1. Decide what you want to accomplish (your long-term **goal**).

2. Determine the necessary **steps** to accomplish this goal.

3. Start making short-term **action plans** with yourself.

4. **Carry out** your action plan.

5. **Check** the results.

6. Make midcourse **corrections** as needed.

Goals

Deciding what you want to accomplish may be the easiest part of being a manager. Think of all the things you would like to do. One of our self-managers wanted to climb twenty steps to her daughter's home so she could join her family for a holiday meal. Another wanted to lose weight so he could receive a hip replacement. Still another wanted to be more socially active. In each case, the goal was one that would take several weeks or even months to accomplish. In fact, one of the problems with goals is they often seem more like dreams. They are so far off that we don't even try to accomplish them. However, a good management program starts (but does not end) with goals. Take a moment now to write your goals on a separate sheet of paper.

Steps

There are many different ways to reach any specific goal. For example, our self-manager who wanted to climb twenty steps could start off with a slow-walking program, knee-strengthening exercises, learning how to use a cane, or starting to climb a few stairs each day. The man who wanted to lose weight could decide to not eat between meals, give up desserts, cut down on fried foods, or start an exercise program. The self-manager who wanted more social contact could find out about community college classes, church groups, or other organizations; call or write friends; or maybe find out about organized trips. She could call the Arthritis Foundation, Arthritis Society, or Arthritis Care to find out about support groups, exercise classes, or volunteer opportunities.

As you can see, there are many options for reaching each goal. The job here is to list the options and then choose one or two on which you would like to work. Write the options for each of your goals on a separate sheet of paper. Put a star next to those on which you would like to work: If you cannot think of any options, share your goal with friends, family, or health professionals and ask for suggestions. Remember, self-managers use consultants.

Action Plans

A short-term action plan calls for a specific action that you can realistically expect to accomplish within the next week. This is probably your most important self-management tool. Most of us can do things that would make us healthier but often fail to do them. For example, most people with arthritis can walk: some just across the room, others for half a block. Most can walk several blocks, and some can walk a mile (1.5 km) or more. However, few people have a systematic exercise program, even though they know it would be good for them. An action plan helps us to do the things we know we should.

Let's go through all the steps for making a realistic action plan. This is a very important skill and may well determine the success of your self-management program.

First, decide what you will do this week. For our step climber, this might be climbing three steps on four days.

The man trying to lose weight might decide to not eat between meals for three days or to eat chocolate no more than twice a week. This action must be something that you want to do, that you feel you realistically can do, and that is a step on the way to your long-term goal.

Then make a specific plan. This is the most difficult and important part of making an action plan. Deciding what you want to do is worthless without a plan to do it. The plan should contain all of the following steps.

1. Exactly what is it that you are going to do? For example: How far will you walk? How will you eat less? What pain-management technique will you practice?

2. How much will you do? For example: walk around the block; walk for fifteen minutes; climb three stairs; write letters to two friends.

3. When will you do this? Again, this must be specific: before lunch; in the shower; when I come home from work. Connecting a new activity with an old habit is a good way to be sure it gets done.

4. How often will you do the activity? This is a bit tricky. We would all like to do things every day. However, we are human and this is not always possible. It is usually best to make an action plan to do something three or four times a week. If you do more, so much the better. However, if you are like most of us, you can do your activity three or four times and still succeed.

In writing your action plan, there are a couple of guidelines that may help you toward success. First, start where you are or start slowly. If you can walk around the block, start your walking program with walking around the block, not with walking a kilometer or a mile. If you have never done any exercise, start with just a few minutes of warm-up, endurance, and cool-down exercises. A total of five to ten minutes is enough. Some people may start by walking one minute an hour. If you want to lose weight, set a goal based on your eating behaviors, such as not eating after dinner. See Chapter 9 for help in starting an exercise program and Chapter 13 for more information on healthy eating.

Also, give yourself some time off. All people have days when they don't feel like doing anything. Therefore, it is best to say that you will do something three to five times a week but not every day. That way, if you don't feel like walking one day, you can still accomplish your action plan.

Once you've made your action plan, ask yourself the following question: "On a scale of 0 to 10, with 0 being totally unsure and 10 being totally confident, how confident am I that I can complete my action plan?"

If your answer is 7 or above, this is probably a realistic plan. Congratulate yourself; you have done the hard work. If your answer is below 7, then you should reassess your action plan. Ask yourself what makes you uncertain. What problems do you foresee? Then see if you can either solve the problems or change your action plan to make yourself more confident of success.

Once you have made an action plan you are happy with, write it down on an action plan form or calendar and post this sheet where you will see it every day. Keep track of how you are doing and the problems you encounter.

Carrying Out Your Action Plan

If the action plan is well written and realistic, fulfilling it is generally pretty easy. Ask family or friends to check with you on how you are doing. Having to report your progress is good motivation. While carrying out your plan, keep track of your daily activities. All good managers have lists of what they want to accomplish and check things off as they are completed. This will give you guidance on how realistic your planning was, and it will also be useful in making future plans. Make daily notes, even of the things you don't understand at the time. Later, these notes may be useful in establishing a pattern that can be used for problem solving.

For example, our stair-climbing friend never did her climbing. Each day, she had a different problem: not having enough time, being tired, the weather being too cold, and so on. When she looked back, she began to realize that the real problem was that she was afraid that she might fall with no one around to help her. She then decided to use a cane while climbing stairs and to do her climbing when a friend or neighbor was around.

Checking the Results

At the end of each week, see if you are any nearer to accomplishing your goal. Are you able to walk farther? Have you lost weight? Are you less fatigued? Taking stock is important. You may not see progress day by day, but you should see a little progress each week. If your action plan involves exercise, you can use some of the self-tests in chapters 10–12. Also, at the end of each week, check on how well you have fulfilled your action plan. If you are having problems, this is a good time to use consultants. Depending on the problem, consultants may be friends, family, or members of your health-care team. Remember, consultants never solve your problems. They only help you accomplish your goal.

Corrections

In any business, the first plan is not always the workable plan. If something doesn't work, don't give up. Try something else. Modify your short-term plans so that your steps are easier. Give yourself more time to accomplish difficult tasks. Choose new steps to your goal, or check with your consultants for their advice and aid.

If you run into problems, don't stop; get help. For example, one self-manager we know was going to walk with a coworker every day at lunch. The problem was that even though the coworker tried to slow down, she walked too fast. The solution was simple. The woman asked her coworker to always walk slightly behind her. Thus, the self-manager set the pace and was able to continue on her daily walk.

Another self-manager wanted to tell her grown children that hosting big holiday dinners had become too much for her. However, she didn't know how to do this. By talking to friends, she first decided to offer to cook the turkey and have the children each bring a dish and clean up. Then, she rehearsed saying, "I know how much of a tradition holiday dinners are. However, I just can't do as much anymore. I'll cook the turkey, and will you each bring something?" This story had a happy ending because the children had all wanted to help for years but had not offered for fear of offending their mother. Chapters 14–16 can help you with problem management.

For some problems, consultants can be most helpful. If medications are causing problems, ask the advice of your physician. If you just stop taking the drug, you are cheating yourself in two ways. First, you are not getting the benefits of medication. Second, you have not supplied your consultant with the vital information he or she needs to help you manage successfully.

If you really enjoy swimming but have problems because you cannot comfortably turn your head, check with an occupational therapist. You probably don't need ongoing treatment, but one problem-solving visit with a professional may keep you in the water. (In this case, the solution might be a face mask and snorkel.)

The best part of being a good self-manager is the rewards you will get in accomplishing your goals. However, don't wait until your goal is attained; reward yourself frequently. For example, decide that you won't read the paper or watch TV until after you exercise. Thus, these become your reward. One self-manager (she is one of this book's authors) buys only one or two pieces of fruit at a time and walks the half mile to the supermarket every day or two to get more fruit. Rewards don't have to be fancy or expensive, just something that is pleasant and meaningful in your life.

To review, a successful arthritis self-manager does the following:

1. Sets goals

2. Determines what is necessary to reach the goal

3. Makes short-term action plans

4. Carries out the action plans

5. Checks on progress weekly

6. Makes midcourse corrections as necessary

Part III

Hints, Tips, Gadgets, and Resources

Chapter 7

Outsmarting Arthritis

Problem Solving for Success

People who live successfully with arthritis develop ways to make their daily lives easier. They work around problems, create manageable schedules, plan ahead, and try out tips that simplify difficult or painful tasks. Sometimes trying a task in a new way can accidentally make life with arthritis easier. There are times, however, when a new problem comes up or a recurrent problem becomes more bothersome and usual methods don't solve the problem. The activity could be anything: managing your hair, cleaning out the vegetable bins of your refrigerator, traveling abroad, gardening, or playing golf. When pain, stiffness, fatigue, or other factors interfere or prevent you from performing important activities, it is time to take extra steps to solve the problem. If the activity is really important to you, something that you enjoy or value, using a problem-solving approach can help you find a way to do that activity.

Ingredients for Successful Problem Solving

Here are the common elements that might guide you in solving problems of your own.

1. Work on a specific problem that is really important to you to address *now*.

   Target a problem you are having in the context of a specific situation—a problem that is interfering with an important activity in your life. This will make your problem-solving process very concrete and focused. The passion to pursue important activities, wishes, and dreams can be an important impetus to problem solving.

2. Explore the problem to understand its possible causes.

Sometimes there is more to the problem than you think. You can explore a problem in many ways: by practicing parts of the task or visualizing them to try to figure out why they are hard for you, by keeping an open-minded attitude, by anticipating parts of the activity that might be hard for you, or by trying alternate ways to do an activity. Continuing to explore the problem, and keeping an open mind regarding what the problem entails, will allow you to understand and then solve the problem.

3. Experiment with a variety of possible solutions.

Solving a difficult problem usually involves some struggle. Trying a variety of possible solutions has many benefits. You will experience less frustration if one idea fails, and sometimes a combination of solutions solves the problem best. Try different solutions and evaluate the success of each.

Using Resources

Don't forget to use yourself as a resource. Sometimes people immediately embrace the advice of others and minimize their own ideas. Give the problem some thought, and try out some of your own ideas before you ask others for help. More often than not, you will be able to solve much of the problem yourself. If you have done your best to think through a problem on your own, getting input from others and using resources can be invaluable.

Working on Your Own Problem

Now it's your turn to work on an important problem of your own. If you don't have an idea right now, take some time to think about your problem, and come back to this section when you do.

Use the rest of this chapter and the following chapter to get ideas that may help you solve problems that are important to you. Solving problems now may also play a role in preventing future problems by showing you how to get the task done with the least amount of effort. Use your ingenuity to take advantage of the information throughout the rest of this book and from other resources to help you solve problems that are important to you.

Body Mechanics for Home and Office

The principle of body mechanics is to use your muscles and joints efficiently in order to reduce stress, pain, and fatigue. Good joint care occurs when your joints are in good alignment; there is less stress and pressure on joints and the body is better able to absorb shock. Therefore, proper attention to principles of body mechanics can prevent many potential problems.

1. Distribute the Load Over Stronger Joint(s), a Larger Surface Area, or Both

Purposes

▼ To reduce joint stress and prevent joint pain by spreading the weight of objects you are carrying, pushing, or pulling.

▼ To eliminate tight grasping and pinching, since these actions may stress your knuckles or cause hand stiffness. If you notice deformities developing in your hand, ask your doctor about consultation with an occupational therapist. A management program can be developed to meet your specific needs.

Examples

▼ Instead of using your fingers, use the palms of your hands, your forearms, or your elbows.

▼ Instead of your arms, use your whole body. Instead of your back, use your legs.

▼ Use a sponge instead of a dishrag to mop up tables and counters. The water can be squeezed out of the sponge more easily by putting it in the sink and pressing down with your flattened hand.

▼ Hold objects close to your body to reduce the load. This in turn reduces fatigue and joint stress. Objects feel heavier if held farther away from your body and lighter when held closer.

▼ When using spray cans or bottles, push down with the side of the hand instead of the fingertips. When that doesn't work, consider adaptive equipment that will reduce pressure on your hands.

▼ Close plastic containers with your elbow.

▼ Wring out wet washcloths or laundry by wrapping the item over the faucet and squeezing excess water out between the palms of your hands. An alternative is to wrap the item in a thick towel and let the towel soak up the excess moisture.

▼ Spare your hands from difficult-to-open refrigerator doors or cupboards by placing a strap on the handle. To open, simply place your forearm through the strap and pull.

▼ Instead of holding the handles of a rolling pin, place hands flat on top and roll beneath your hands.

▼ When pushing up from a chair, keep your hands facing palm down.

▼ Use your hip to close kitchen or dresser drawers.

▼ Use both arms to take down or hang clothes in the closet.

▼ Instead of placing your fingers through the handle of a coffe cup, encircle it with both hands. Mugs are especially good for this. Try cups and glasses with dif-

A Word About Walking Sticks

One way to relieve hip or knee pain is to use a cane or walking stick. The handle of the cane should reach your wrist when your hand is at your side. To make the cane more stable, buy a wide rubber tip at any pharmacy. The tip on most canes is too narrow.

To use a cane, put it in the hand opposite your bad side: if your left hip hurts, hold your cane in your right hand. When your left foot is forward, your cane should also be forward. By distributing your weight in this way, you relieve some of the pressure on your hip.

Unfortunately, some people are too proud to use a cane. They think it shows weakness or that they are old. Nothing could be further from the truth. Using a cane shows you are smart and confident enough to do what is best for you.

Canes can also be very stylish. Look around and get a lucite cane, a colored cane, or a fancy cane handle. A cane can be dressed up with a scarf or fancy tape. Some of our self-managers have a whole collection of canes, from walking sticks for picnics to black shiny canes with silver handles for formal affairs.

ferent shapes and textures to find out what works best for you.

▼ Carry your plate back to the kitchen by "scooping" it up with the palms of both hands.

▼ When carrying a briefcase, use a shoulder strap and avoid using the handles. Carry a purse on your forearm or use a shoulder bag and avoid clutching it in your hand.

▼ Holding a grocery bag close to your body with both arms makes it feel lighter and reduces fatigue and joint stress.

▼ A book holder or pillow on your lap serves to support a book and frees your hands.

2. Avoid Maintaining the Same Joint Position for Prolonged Periods

Purposes

▼ To reduce joint stiffness.

▼ To prevent joint contractures.

Examples

▼ **Hips and Knees:** Alternate between sitting and standing positions. Although the sitting position is generally recommended to reduce stress on the lower joints and prevent fatigue, it is important to get up and stretch frequently.

▼ **Knees:** When sitting, change the position of your legs so that your knees are periodically stretched out. This can reduce knee stiffness and pain when you return to standing.

▼ **Ankles:** Flex and point your toes while watching television or talking with a friend. You don't have to wait for a specific exercise time to do your stretching exercises (see Chapter 10).

▼ **Hands:** Avoid sustained grasps on objects. For example, take rest breaks when you are writing or cooking. Consider alternating writing tasks with computer activities.

3. Reduce Excess Body Weight

Purpose

▼ To reduce stress on joints and fatigue.

4. Use Good Posture

Purpose

▼ To use your muscles and joints more efficiently. Proper body alignment when standing, sitting, lifting, and changing positions accomplishes this.

Standing

Good posture means that the three curves of your spine—neck, middle back, and low back—are gentle and small. These gentle curves provide stability and absorb shock when you walk and move. If you stand in a military posture with your chest puffed out, you will flatten the middle curve of your back. If you are extremely round shouldered, you will exaggerate the middle curve of your back. If you stand with a swayback, you will exaggerate the lower curve in your back. When curves are exaggerated or eliminated, the spine becomes less effective as a shock absorber and strain and pain are more likely.

Check your posture using the checklist on page 59 to identify strengths and weaknesses. Look in a mirror or ask a friend to help you.

Standing Posture Checklist

▼ Ears directly over your shoulders

▼ Shoulders the same height and relaxed (Rounding your shoulders and bringing your head too far forward are common posture mistakes. This position can cause neck and upper-back pain.)

▼ Shoulders in line with your hips

▼ Stomach muscles lightly contracted

▼ Hips in line with your knees and feet

▼ Knees straight but unlocked (Avoid locking your knees, as this puts increased strain on your lower back.)

▼ Feet shoulder-width apart (A plumb line dropped from the top of the head would pass through the ear, shoulder, hip, knee, and ankle.)

▼ Even weight on both feet (Placing one foot on a footstool helps to reduce back strain during activities that are performed in one position.)

Sitting Posture Checklist

▼ Head over shoulders

▼ Shoulders relaxed, not elevated (raise your shoulders up to your ears and then relax them to make sure they are not elevated)

▼ Upper back relaxed and over hips

▼ Knees even with hips

▼ Buttocks flat on seat

▼ Feet flat on floor or footrest

▼ Even weight on both hips

▼ When sitting at a computer work-station, position your keyboard so that your wrists are in the neutral (natural resting) position* and your elbows are bent at waist height when you type. Select a chair that is comfortable and encourages correct posture. If needed, add a small pillow to support your lower back and a footrest to support your feet.

▼ When working at your workbench or in the kitchen, a bar-height stool with footrest allows you to sit while you work on projects, wash dishes, or prepare meals. This helps to prevent fatigue, as well as providing a suitable work height.

The posture checklists above focus on ideal posture. If you already know you cannot achieve "ideal" posture because of body changes or long-standing bad posture habits, try the Natural Posture Test (page 62). It is designed to help you find the best posture for your body. Forcing your body into a painful position will not benefit you. Alternatively, maintaining the best alignment that is comfortable for you reduces strain on your muscles and joints.

Standing Up

1. Scoot forward in your chair so that you are near the edge.

2. Place one foot slightly in front of the other so that it is directly under the knee. The other foot is behind the knee. Avoid putting too much pressure on your hands.

---

* To find the neutral or natural resting wrist position, put your forearm and hand on a table. The forearm is flat but the palm cups. The wrist is not exactly straight but bends slightly upward.

3. Exhale as you come up to increase ease. If you have a hard time coming to stand, consider gently rocking back and forth three times to give you some momentum. Chairs that are several inches higher than normal, either through the use of pillows or chair leg extenders, make it easier to stand up.

Lifting

To lift objects from the ground or low shelves, bend your legs instead of your back; pick up the object, holding it as close to your body as possible; and rise, letting your leg muscles do the work.

People with knee problems may want to let someone else lift heavy objects, since the knees are strained from the weight of the object as well as from their own body weight. People with knee and hip problems who need to lift objects may benefit from consulting a physical therapist for alternative methods.

Getting Up from the Floor

1. Roll onto one side.

2. With the upper hand, push yourself up enough to get your lower elbow under you.

3. Walk up to sitting using your hands.

4. Reach across your body until both hands are on the floor at one side.

5. Shift your weight sideways; tuck your knees under and get up onto all fours. If your wrists get painful, come up onto your forearms.

6. Crawl to the nearest steady chair and place your hands on the seat for support.

7. Putting weight onto your hands, bring one knee up and put that foot flat. Bring your stronger leg into this position, ready to push up.

8. Push up with that leg, bearing much of your weight on your hands as they rest on the chair. Consider putting your forearms onto the chair rather than just your hands.

9. When both feet are flat on the floor, begin to straighten your legs. Stop. Keep your head down and let your circulation catch up with the change of position.

10. Now stand up fully straight. But again, stop a moment before you start to walk. Let your circulation adjust. Many people feel faint if they stand up too fast.

Natural Posture Test
This is easiest performed in a chair.

1. Sit in a chair comfortably. Make sure you clear the back of the chair.

2. Slump as far forward as you can. Return to your starting position.

3. Arch your back as much as you can without experiencing pain. Return to your starting posture.

4. Now try to position yourself between your slumped and arched position. This posture should be comfortable. If it is not, make sure to adjust your position.

It is helpful to have a friend or family member present to give you feedback on your posture if possible.

Chairs you sit in regularly have an effect on your posture. Select a chair that:

▼ Has a firm seat

▼ Has a fairly straight back

If you are selecting a chair for a workstation, choose one that:

▼ Has an adjustable backrest height and angle (avoid chairs with S-shaped curves)

▼ Has an adjustable-height seat so that it is the proper height for your work surface

▼ Has casters to allow moving from desktop to computer

▼ Has a rounded end to the seat so that it does not cut into your legs

Efficiency Principles

If you plan and organize your tasks and workspaces you will eliminate unnecessary steps, which saves time and energy. This helps reduce fatigue. Hasty movements yield results no more quickly than organized movements, and they often end in extra work. As the saying goes, "Haste makes waste." Both tension and fatigue are increased when we feel rushed.

1. Plan
Determine the following:

▼ Is the task necessary?

▼ Can the task be simplified?

▼ Who should perform the task?

▼ What steps are involved in completing the task?

▼ In what order will these steps be most efficient?

▼ What is the best time of day or week to perform the task?

▼ Do you need rest periods to complete the task?

▼ What is the best body position to use to complete the task?

Examples

▼ Start large tasks well before the deadline so you can pace yourself: for example, income tax, school papers, bills, greeting cards.

▼ Make entertaining easier. Spread tasks over several days. Select foods that you can prepare ahead of time. Get help for heavy cleaning.

▼ Alternate repetitive cooking tasks such as cutting, chopping, and stirring to reduce stress on your hands. Take short breaks when cooking large quantities. Alternate sitting and standing to reduce fatigue and joint stress.

▼ Buy vegetables and condiments already chopped in the frozen food and produce section of your grocery to simplify cooking. Salad bars at grocery stores are excellent places to purchase fresh, precut vegetables and fruits.

▼ Create a cleaning schedule that works for you. List your regular cleaning tasks. Consider spreading out light cleaning tasks over a week. Schedule one or two heavy cleaning tasks per month. Complete them on a "good day."

▼ Use address and return labels for mail to reduce writing strain.

▼ Combine several errands in one trip whenever possible. If you have to go downstairs or to another part of the house or place of work, try to accomplish several things at a time.

▼ Work on an assembly-line basis. First gather all items you need to complete the task and place them at your workspace. Choose a comfortable position to work, then work in the most efficient order.

2. Organize

Examples

▼ Store equipment and supplies that you use regularly between eye and hip level. This will minimize bending, stooping, and needless searching. Store the heavier items in easy reach, such as on countertops.

▼ Use kitchen and office organizers, such as bins, dividers, turntables, pull-out shelves, and spice racks, to locate items quickly.

▼ Store items in the locations where they are most frequently used.

▼ Eliminate clutter. Remove unnecessary or infrequently used items from shelves.

▼ To remove clutter: Put items you do not use in a bin; if you do not look for these in a month, get rid of them. If you have a very cluttered area, put away one item every time you pass by. Clutter does not have to be organized all at one time.

▼ Put duplicates of inexpensive items, such as cleaners, scissors, and cellophane tape, in all the places where they are regularly used.

▼ Use special organizers for closets to maximize your use of space.

▼ Store seasonal items, such as winter hats and scarves, in clear plastic containers so they are easy to locate.

3. Balance Work with Rest

One of the most effective means of avoiding fatigue is to schedule short but frequent rest periods throughout the day. One way of resting muscles is to use other ones. For example, after sitting, stand up and stretch. After an extended time in one posture, go into an alternate posture to relieve overused joints and muscles. If you can prevent fatigue, even if it means stopping in the middle of a job, your endurance over the long run will be increased. While stopping to rest is difficult, remember that long work periods require longer recovery periods.

Examples

▼ Schedule frequent rest periods throughout the day. These will vary for each individual. An example might be to rest ten minutes out of every hour, instead of working for three hours straight. Even a short break is better than none.

▼ Alternate heavy and light work tasks during each day. In addition, plan the more difficult or lengthy tasks when you know you have the endurance to do them.

▼ Sitting to work is a form of rest since it uses less energy than standing. However, if you spend your workday behind a desk, you will find that moving around at regular intervals keeps you more alert and energetic.

Product-Selection Principles

These principles help you choose new products and evaluate those you already own. Using products with the features described in this section helps reduce joint stress, pain, and fatigue by allowing you to complete a task with the least amount of effort.

If you need information about finding any of these items, call your Arthritis Foundation or Arthritis Society chapter or contact the occupational therapy department at your local hospital.

1. Use Wheels

Purposes

▼ To reduce friction, lessening the resistance between surfaces.

▼ To avoid lifting and carrying.

Examples

▼ Use a cart or attach a carrier with wheels to items to avoid the strain of carrying.

▼ Use wheels to transport. Utility carts, tea tables, and shopping carts are just a few examples of readily available items on wheels.

▼ Use a luggage carrier or suitcase on wheels when traveling. This allows you to take most of the strain off your arms as you push or pull the suitcase. Consider using small luggage even to tote crafts or papers.

▼ Special key-holders allow you to turn a key by holding the handle in the palm of your hand. These are available through special equipment vendors or can be made by riveting a piece of wood or metal to the key.

2. Use Extended Handles

Purpose

▼ Products with long handles or long attachments let you use less force to manipulate objects. These products help conserve strength.

Examples

▼ A piece of wood, metal, or firm plastic can be attached to many types of objects to increase the length of the handle.

Lightweight Options For Everyday Objects

Item	Lightweight Options	What To Avoid
Dishes	plastic; Corelle	stoneware
Pots/pans	stainless steel with black stay-cool handles	cast iron
Bowls	plastic; aluminum	Pyrex; stoneware
Baking dishes and casseroles	foil pans; aluminum; microwave cookware; Farberware; T-fal	Corningware
Luggage/ briefcases	nylon; canvas	leather; hardback
Fans	plastic	metal
Winter coats	fiberfill; goose down	leather; wool

3. Use Lightweight Objects

Purpose

▼ To reduce joint stress, pain, and fatigue.

Examples

▼ Lightweight objects are easier to carry and to clean. The table above lists a few examples of lightweight alternative products.

4. Use Large Handles

Purposes

▼ To help maintain a secure hold when hands are weak.

▼ To help hold an object if fingers do not fully close.

▼ To lessen tension required to maintain your hold on objects.

Examples

▼ Purchase silverware, pens, tools, kitchen utensils, and so on, that are made with bulky handles about one inch (2.5 cm) in diameter.

▼ Build up utensil handles. Pipe-insulation tubing with an opening from 3/8 to 3/4 inch (1 to 2 cm) in diameter offers an easy and inexpensive way to do this. You may need to tape the slit in the tubing shut. Most hardware stores sell pipe-insulation tubing in four-foot (1.2 m) lengths at reasonable prices.

▼ Purchase pencil grips from office supply stores or order them from daily living equipment catalogues or buy pens with built-in grips.

▼ A doorknob extender allows you to open the door with the palm of the hand instead of with the fingers.

▼ Open a car door with an aid in the palm of your hand.

▼ Attach a dowel or a piece of wood to a can opener and hold on to this lengthened handle when opening cans. Never use a butterfly can opener. The pressure required to operate one is extreme; use an electric or wall-mounted type.

▼ Open flip-top cans with a table knife.

▼ Foam padding added to such articles as a toothbrush, pen, razor, fork, or comb increases the size of the handle.

5. Use Convenience Items

Purposes

▼ To decrease the length of time and number of steps needed to complete a task.

▼ To reduce joint stress and pain and fatigue.

Examples

▼ Use labor-saving devices such as a food processor, blender, microwave, electric toothbrush, and electric hedger.

▼ Purchase permanent press clothing.

Chapter 8

Self-Helpers: 100+ Hints and Aids

The preceding chapter, "Outsmarting Arthritis," provided you with basic principles and examples of how to use your joints appropriately. Additional hints are provided in this chapter, not only on how to use your joints, but also on how to perform activities if your general mobility or finger coordination is impaired.

You may find that you are already doing many of the things mentioned in this chapter. It is true that necessity is the mother of invention. If you combine your needs and your common sense, you will probably come up with another hundred hints. Use the suggestions here as a springboard for additional ideas for making your life easier and more comfortable. Then share them with friends and others who might benefit from them.

Dressing

If buttons are difficult to manipulate, sew Velcro on clothing. Attach buttons permanently to the top side of the garment, and use the Velcro as a fastener. Velcro can be found in most sewing stores.

An alternative to buttons on sleeves is elasticized thread sewn on button cuffs. This often provides sufficient give for your hands to slide through.

In the future, buy clothes that are easy to put on and easy to care for. Tops should be large enough or designed so that sleeves are easy to slip into—you may want to avoid turtlenecks. Elastic waistbands around pants should be loose enough to slip easily over hips. Fastenings should be located in the front and be easy to manipulate.

If reaching the clothes in the closet is difficult, have someone lower the rod.

Special devices to assist with shoes include long-handled shoehorns, elastic shoelaces, and zipper laces. Velcro can be useful for fastening shoes as well as clothing.

A bent coat hanger, reacher, or dressing stick can assist with pulling pants up, straightening shirts, or retrieving clothes slightly out of reach.

Place large rings, thread, or leather hoops on zipper tabs.

Fasten your bra in front of you. Turn bra around and pull it into place. Try front-closure bras.

Buttonhooks work well to fasten buttons. You can make your own buttonhook with a six-inch (15 cm) piece of wooden dowel and a large paper clip.

Shoes
When buying shoes, look for the following features:

▼ Low heel or wedge, no higher than one inch (2.5 cm)

▼ Toe area wide and deep enough to prevent rubbing or crunching of toes

▼ Cushioned sole to pad the ball of your foot; avoid wooden soles

▼ Laces, buckles, or Velcro to loosen or tighten when feet swell

▼ Soft upper material to give or be stretched to relieve pressure on specific areas

Don't rule out gym shoes. Many running, walking, and aerobic shoes meet the above criteria. Some now have Velcro closures. If your present shoes have the recommended characteristics but are still uncomfortable, consult your physician or podiatrist.

A sock aid will allow you to put on your socks if you cannot reach your feet. First, you need to slide your sock onto the sock aid shell. Then drop the sock aid to the floor. Slide your foot into the shell and pull the sock on gently with the long handles. You can make your own sock aid by cutting X-ray film or construction board into the shape of an upside-down "ten-gallon hat" and attaching a piece of cord through a hole punched in each side of the hat's "brim."

A variety of shoe adaptations are available at regular stores and orthopedic shoe stores or can be custom made by orthotists. Orthotists are professionals who custom make and custom fit special equipment based on a referral from a physician. For example, they make braces, cervical collars, and footwear adaptations. Following are some common shoe adaptations:

▼ Gel soles

▼ Soft-cushion inserts

▼ Custom-molded inserts

▼ Pads for ball of foot

▼ External bar under shoe

To help heel pain, tighten the lower part of the shoe laces. For men's shoes, try two shoelaces, tight on the bottom, looser on top.

Talk with your doctor about exercises to stretch your calf as another way to help.

Most of the items above take pressure off the ball of the foot. Consult your physician or podiatrist when choosing the proper adaptation for you. Foot problems are very individual.

New shoes and shoe adaptations can alter your walking pattern. Wear them in gradually, increasing time increments starting with thirty minutes or less to avoid pain. It is surprising how much pain new footwear can cause when it is not introduced gradually. If you purchase custom-made equipment, make sure to ask for a wearing schedule.

Bathing and Hygiene

A long-handled sponge or brush can be used to soap yourself when bathing.

Tub and shower benches, or a webbed plastic lawn chair, allow you to sit while showering, which helps prevent fatigue. The benches also provide a place to sit when getting down into the tub is difficult.

Safety considerations when bathing include the use of nonskid safety strips or a rubber bathmat on the tub bottom. In addition, grab bars can be permanently installed on the wall or attached to the edge of the bathtub.

A removable showerhead with a long hose makes rinsing easier.

Grab bars provide a safe hold when you are climbing in and out of the tub or shower and also provide a place to pull or push up from when you are in the tub.

A bath mitt can be bought or easily made by sewing two facecloths together. Lather it up and soap yourself the easy way.

After bathing, put on a terry robe and let it soak up the water as you pat yourself dry. This lets you avoid the sometimes painful motions needed to towel yourself dry.

Use a shower caddy to keep soap and shampoo within easy reach.

Special long-handled combs and brushes are useful when shoulder and elbow limitations prevent you from reaching your head. Consider a short "wash and wear" haircut for increased ease.

The Freshette Director makes it possible for women to urinate while standing. It is a part of a complete portable restroom system that can be used standing, sitting in a chair, or lying in bed.

A raised toilet seat or commode over the toilet provides greater height and thus makes standing up easier.

In addition, a toilet safety frame or a grab bar installed on the wall next to the toilet will allow you to use your arms when sitting and standing. You can also now purchase toilets that are several inches higher than usual, so you might consider replacing your toilet.

Electric toothbrushes and Water Piks make oral hygiene easier. In addition, there is a device that holds dental floss, allowing you to floss your teeth with one hand holding onto the handle; ask your dentist about these or check your local drugstore.

Put foam curlers onto eyeliner and mascara handles for better grip.

Use the heel of your hand to squeeze the toothpaste tube or press down on a toothpaste pump.

For feminine hygiene, wind tampon string around a pencil. Keep the pencil horizontal, and pull gently with both hands for easier removal. Some brands of tampons have loops rather than straight strings, with which you can more easily use a pencil or your fingers to pull. For those who use pads, a detachable shower hose with an adjustable spray may be useful for more thorough genital-area cleaning.

Enlarge the handle of a razor by adding pipe-insulation tubing or by taping a small sponge around the handle.

Ask family members to fold the end of the toilet paper into a V. This makes the paper easier to grasp.

Cooking

Microwave ovens save time and energy. They are easy to operate, easy to clean, and usually easy to reach since they are often placed on countertops.

To avoid lifting pots heavy with food and the water the food was boiled in, consider several alternatives. One is to place a frying basket inside a pot so you can lift the food out with the basket and discard the water later. Spaghetti cookers come with a perforated insert and can serve in the same manner. Or you may want to ladle the contents out.

To open jars, install a jar opener that will grip the lid as you use both hands to turn the jar itself. Also, ask other members of the family not to close lids too tightly.

Use lightweight cooking utensils, bowls, and dishes. Avoid cast-iron skillets and heavy ceramic bowls.

Select appliances with levers or push buttons that are easy to operate.

Store canned goods so that the same items are lined up behind one another. This way you can tell from the front label what is in the back of the shelf.

Plan and prepare meals ahead of time to avoid last-minute preparations. Cook enough so you have leftovers to reheat the next day. Also, try preparing double or triple portions and freezing the extra.

Find dishes that require minimal preparation and little effort. Today many convenience foods, ready mixes, and frozen foods contain low salt, low fat, and minimal additives.

One-pot meals require less cleanup.

Serve foods in the same containers in which they were cooked. Use casseroles, Farberware, and other lightweight attractive cooking vessels.

Use throwaway pie tins and other disposable utensils to cut down on dishwashing.

Line pans with aluminum foil for easier cleanup.

Use cookie sheets and pans with special surfaces that prevent sticking and messy cleanup, spray them with a nonstick product, or line them with parchment paper.

Mixing bowls can be stabilized by placing them on a wet washcloth or on little octopus-like suction cups. You can also place a bowl in a drawer at work height.

Place small amounts of flour and sugar in containers so you can scoop out the amount needed and avoid lifting heavy bags each time.

Mitt pot holders allow you to lift hot pans with the palms of both hands.

Attach a spray hose at the kitchen sink so that you can fill pots with water on the countertop. Slide pots to the stove to avoid lifting.

Try using a pizza wheel instead of a knife to cut various foods.

Food processors make food preparation a snap, especially when large quantities of food must be chopped, sliced, or grated.

If you cannot afford an electric food processor, use an onion chopper.

You can cut with your wrist in a neutral position using an ergonomic knife or a pizza cutter. They are available in a variety of sizes and styles.

When peeling vegetables, try a commercial peeler with a wide handle, such as the Good Grips peelers by OXO, or build up the handle of a standard peeler.

Use a pot with a wet cloth draped over it as a support for a bowl when pouring batter into a baking pan.

Entertaining

Arrange a buffet meal. Let your guests select their own silver, plates, and napkins and serve themselves from large dishes of food.

Use nice paper plates and plastic utensils to eliminate dishwashing.

Have a potluck meal, where each guest brings a dish of food or some paper goods.

Housekeeping

Keep a set of cleaning supplies in each area where they are used, to eliminate needless walking.

To clean the bathtub, sit on a low stool next to the tub and use a long-handled sponge.

Long-handled sponges can also be used to clean around door sills and other hard-to-reach places.

Use a long-handled dustpan and small broom to clean up dry spills from floors.

Use an adjustable-height ironing board so that you can sit to iron. Attach a cord-minder to keep the cord out of your way.

Carpeting or foam-backed rugs help to ease ankle and foot pain when prolonged standing and moving about are necessary.

Use gravity whenever possible. Let your clothes fall from the dryer into the basket. When scooping them out, you may want to use a reacher or stick.

Laundry bags that were originally intended for washing delicate items like nylons can be used for all small pieces of clothing (socks, underwear) and thus eliminate searching in the machine.

If lifting a heavy detergent box is difficult, you can either have someone else pour some detergent into a smaller container or scoop rather than pour detergent. Liquid detergents may also be more manageable.

Try using the old-style push-on clothespins rather than pinch clothespins.

Front-loading washers are generally easier to use than top-loading washers. Raise the washer on blocks to eliminate bending and make laundering easier.

Consider computer shopping services if it is hard for you to get to the store.

Call your local grocery to find out whether they deliver at an affordable price. Sometimes a local teenager can shop for you more economically. Also, local villages, cities, or townships can often be a resource for transportation to the store.

Use lockable casters on furniture. It will be easier to move when cleaning. These allow you to roll the furniture when you wish but they lock in place for everyday use.

Use a large spatula or an oven shovel to tuck in sheets.

The touch-tronic is a device that allows you to turn lamps on and off by touching them with your fingers or adding a slide switch. Contact your local lighting store to order it and to learn about different options.

Enlarged knobs are available to place on lamps as well as appliances such as washing machines (certain brands only) to increase ease of handling. Check with your washing machine manufacturer if the controls are difficult to operate.

Child Care

Be sure to test out car seats, strollers, cribs and other equipment before you buy them. Explore the variety of lightweight equipment available for infants. Take advantage of carriers and strollers designed to hold infant car seats.

Take good care of yourself. To avoid repeatedly lifting your baby in and out of the car consider asking a family member or a caretaker to watch your child while you run multiple errands. Consider scheduling a nap for yourself every day, and make it a priority. When your role feels overwhelming, get help from those around you and express appreciation for that help. Treat yourself to a massage now and then. Make sure to find someone who is experienced in working with people who have arthritis or fibromyalgia.

If you are having trouble getting your child from your lap onto the floor consider a slide down transfer. Ask the child to roll onto her stomach and slide down your leg. This technique is useful for children six months or older (prior to six months babies do not have sufficient head control). Be innovative in finding ways to pick up your child. When she is standing and walking, scooping her with one hand on the legs and the other on the back is easier on the hands and wrists than lifting from under the arms. Once your child can walk or crawl up stairs, let her do the work and spot her as she climbs.

Consider placing a piece of equipment on wheels—for example, a stroller or highchair—in every room to help you transport the baby when you are tired.

Work with your baby to teach her to not wiggle during diapering and dressing. Consider distracting your young child with laughter and funny voices to help with wiggling during tasks such as washing hair. Try a different position for diapering such as rolling the baby on her side. Alternatively, teach the baby to help you by tapping her buttocks while you say "up" and then slide the diaper under her.

Select baby clothes that are easy to take on and off, such as clothes that stretch and clothes that slip on overhead. Clothes a size or half size too big are easier to get on and off. Look for generous neck openings to make dressing easier. Test out buttons, snaps, and so on to find out which are easiest for you. Use Velcro fasteners when possible.

Warm water soaks for sore hands or body parts can be a big help in dealing with the demands of parenthood. Some people respond better to cool water soaks or alternating warm and cool water.

Build up the handle of a spoon for yourself and use another for baby.

It is especially important to use good posture when picking up and breast-feeding your child. Many parents carry their child on one side of their body and can eventually experience pain related to the body's "unevenness." Try to pick up and carry your child on both sides of your body, if this is possible. Take the time to position your baby when breastfeeding; use a pillow thick enough to bring your baby to you.

Find ways to play that work for you. If holding your child is hard, you can tease and play in a bed pushed against the wall while the child lies on her side. Singing songs, listening to music, reading books, watching a favorite video are all ways to play and relate. Think about ways to play when you are tired. Just cuddling together while lying down or sitting close can create a bond. What is most important is feeling close to your child and making a connection.

Picking up toys can be a challenge. Consider using a reacher (two-foot-long piece of equipment with a gripper at the end) to pick up light items. Hire a mother's helper to play fetch or other games that you cannot play with your child.

Store toys and books at a level your child can reach. Keep a limited number of toys available to avoid excessive pickup and cleanup. Rotate toys to keep it interesting for your child.

On a bad day, it is important to explain to your young child that your pain, fatigue, irritability, stiffness, or other unpleasant symptom has nothing to do with him. Consider using relaxation and pain relief techniques such as deep breathing mentioned in Chapter 14 to help you manage your symptoms.

Create a rhythm to your life. Plan a regular schedule for some routine tasks such as clothes shopping, grocery shopping, cooking, cleaning, and laundry. If you visit a few friends or relatives regularly, store a small supply of clothes, diapers, wipes, and other needs at their house so you carry less. At home, keep supplies at every location that you use them. So if you dress the baby in the family room and his room, then keep clothes, diapers, and so on in both locations. Keep the baby's supplies in easy reach for you but out of your baby's reach. Look at the efficiency principles on pages 63–66 for more ideas to make your day-to-day life easier.

You can also create order and rhythm in the household by establishing routines for your child. For example, the morning routine could be get up, go to the bathroom, wash hands, brush teeth, get dressed, and eat breakfast. Offer your child a reward each time he or she completes the routine behaviors. Rewarding positive behavior tends to create more positive behavior. Order in the household creates a calmer and less stressful atmosphere.

There are resources available to provide assistance with adaptive equipment, support from other parents, and help with problem solving. You can contact an occupational therapist in your area, The Parent Empowerment Network, or Through the Looking Glass (see "Resources for Parents" on page 96 for contact information). The Parent Empowerment Network offers online resources for parents with disabilities, adaptive parenting products, a place where parents with all sorts of disabilities can share strategies for independent parenting and child care tasks, and links to other sites with more information. Through the Looking Glass (TLG) is a national resource center that has pioneered research, training, and services for families in which a child, parent, or grandparent has a disability or medical issue. Free services available nationally include information and referral, technical assistance and consultations, professional trainings and workshops, national library and resources clearing house, publications and training modules, parent-to-parent network, international newsletter, website, and bulletin boards. A free newsletter is available about three times a year.

Work

At a computer workstation:

▼ Avoid prolonged use of laptop computers. Because the keyboard is attached to the screen, these encourage poor head and neck posture.

▼ Add a small towel roll behind your lower back if your chair does not provide sufficient support.

▼ Select a document holder that is the same height and distance from you as your screen.

▼ Position your monitor so that the top of the screen is at or just below eye level.

▼ Use a footrest if your feet do not touch the floor.

▼ Consider forearm supports or wrist rests if your chair does not have supportive arms.

▼ Position your arms so that your elbows form a 90-degree angle.

▼ Keep your elbow and wrist in a neutral position (see footnote on page 60), parallel to the floor.

▼ Consider getting a headset if you use the phone while you type or write.

▼ An aerobic mouse allows you to work with your hand, fingers, wrist, and forearm in a position called functional neutral. The arm using the mouse is in a natural position that requires less effort and puts less stress on your muscles and joints; the wrist is in its natural relaxed position. There is an option to buy software that makes it a "clickless" mouse.

▼ Forearm supports move with you as you work at a computer terminal. They reduce strain in the arms, neck, and shoulders by providing additional support. Consider these if you are unable to work at a conventional computer work-station.

▼ An angled work surface encourages good posture during reading and writing tasks. It reduces strain on the neck and upper back.

When writing at a desk, do not lean forward; sit tall and bend the neck only slightly. People with neck problems may want to consider getting a drafting table with an adjustable slant.

If you wear bifocals and have rheumatoid or psoriatic arthritis, do gentle range of motion exercises (pages 121–122) to the neck to prevent stiffness.

Take a break from prolonged sitting, and do exercises to reduce tension, such as Shoulder Rolls (page 126), Two-Way Neck Stretch (page 122), or Hi and Bye (page 130).

If sitting for long periods is uncomfortable and you have the space, set up an additional standing-height workstation by using an adjustable table such as a drafting table. You can use this to alternate between working in sitting and standing positions.

Recreation or Leisure Time

An embroidery frame that can be attached to a table or chair will allow you to do needlework and sewing without using your hands to stabilize the article. These are available primarily through self-help aid catalogs.

If you like to play cards, try using a card holder. These can be purchased through mail-order catalogues or easily made by sawing a slit in a piece of wood. You can also make your own card holder with a box. Simply take the cover off and put it under the box. Your cards can be lined up in the lip of the lid and rest against the box.

Use loop scissors when sewing to avoid pressure and pain on the thumb joint.

Afternoon exercises or sports are a really good way to break up the day. Try to set up a schedule to work such that you can take an extended break to swim or exercise during the lunch hour.

Walking A Dog That Pulls

If you haven't already done so, consider attending a training class to learn to manage and enjoy your animal. Ask about the class philosophy and physical demands of the class before you sign up. Many trainers have their own preferences for training aids, such as head collars, body harnesses, prong collars, and choke collars. Get help in selecting aids and fitting your dog. Some pet stores will fit your dog right in the store. A proper fit is critical. Try out the fasteners to make sure you can manage them yourself. Training aids are designed to be worn only while walking your dog, so make sure you can get them on and off yourself, unless someone is always home to help you.

Head collars work similarly to halters on horses, allowing for gentle control of the head and using the principle that where the nose goes, the body will follow. The Gentle Leader is one popular brand. Body harnesses are used most often for dogs with fragile necks and small dogs but some feel they help with any dog that pulls. Although a prong collar appears cruel and gruesome, many dog trainers feel it is safer and more humane than a choke collar. The prong collar applies even pressure and requires a less forceful and painful correction. The prong collar will only tighten to a fixed endpoint. A snap-on prong collar is easier to fasten than the traditional version. The choke collar has no endpoint and dogs have died from the use of a choke collar. If you choose a choke collar get instructions on how to use it correctly and safely. Sometimes your dog will not accept the collar that seems best for him, so you may have to be flexible in your choices.

If the special leashes are too hard on your hands or too hard to get on your dog, try this simple trick. Run a leather leash along the dog's back. Wrap it around the dog's body immediately in front of his lower legs and pull through to make a loop; it acts as a body harness and helps some dogs mind.

If you build up the handle on a conventional leash, you can use a less forceful grip.

Gardening

Gardening is the perfect opportunity to practice the body mechanic, efficiency principles, and product selection suggestions in the previous chapter. Specifically the following principles apply:

▼ Distribute the load over stronger joints, a larger surface area, or both

▼ Avoid maintaining the same joint position for a prolonged period

▼ Maintain good posture

▼ Plan ahead

▼ Organize

▼ Balance work with rest

▼ Use product selection principles

The body can get a workout during gardening; to minimize soreness, warmup prior to starting and cool down before finishing. You can choose some light stretches from chapters 9–11.

When gardening, try sitting on a small stool instead of kneeling to weed or plant. If you prefer kneeling, consider kneepads or the Easy Kneeler. The Easy Kneeler allows you to lower yourself down and push yourself up with minimal strain. It also can be turned over and used as a seat to work in raised flower beds or planter boxes.

Use gloves to protect your hands. Take advantage of the variety of ergonomic gardening tools made by Fiskars, OXO, Peta, and others. Peta Easy-grip garden tools are designed with an angled handle to keep the hand and wrist in a natural stress-free position, thus preventing strain and making gardening easier.

There is a back-preserver attachment for shovels and a different attachment to be used with hoes and rakes. These tools can easily be attached to your own equipment.

Seek out the latest resources on gardening by searching the web or book venders using descriptors such as "gardening with arthritis," "ergonomic tools," "tools for comfort." One site that contains a wealth of information on gardening, tools, and equipment vendors is the Gardens for Everybody site (see Useful Resources on page 94).

Consider using raised beds or containers for your garden.

Limit lifting, and, when you do lift, remember to use your best body mechanics.

To reduce grasp, consider small plants for flower or vegetable gardens or seed tapes rather than gripping individual seeds.

Driving

When buying a car, look for doors that are easy to open and close, storage that is easy to reach, such as in a hatchback model, and seat adjustment handles that are easy to reach and manipulate.

Attach a loop of fabric to the inside door handle to make the door easier to close.

Auxiliary or wide-angle mirrors allow for increased visibility when neck movement is limited.

To make driving more comfortable and prevent back strain, look into obtaining cushions for the car. You can purchase cushions for the seat back or for the seat itself, to improve posture and prevent slouching. Many cars now come equipped with a lumbar support for the driver. If you use this support, make sure it does not push your back so far forward that it is painful.

Keeping Joints Warm

Use the extra-long heating pads that wrap around an arm or leg and fasten with Velcro to warm an elbow or knee. Use them for up to twenty minutes and then re-move for at least twenty minutes before using them again.

Make your own hot pack. Place rice or beans in a sock and heat in the microwave oven about three min-utes. Put a glass of water in also to prevent damage to your microwave. Remove the sock carefully—it may be very hot—and do not place it directly on bare skin.

Soak stiff, sore, or cold hands in warm water. This is especially useful to loosen them from morning stiffness. At night, warm the hands in this manner: Rub in hand lotion, and wear cotton gloves while sleeping.

Thermoelastic gloves are especially warming be-cause they are made from wool and elastic fibers. They are available in some pharmacies.

Thermoelastic products are also available for knees and elbows, or use a soft, thick kneesock. Cut the sock so you have a tube approximately seven inches (18 cm) long and place the tube over your knee or elbow. Microwavable heat wraps are available for the hand, wrist, knee, elbow, ankle, and torso.

Use electric blankets as a lightweight cover; they are especially useful in warming the bed before you get into it.

An alternative way to stay warm during the night or when resting is to sleep inside a sleeping bag that is placed under a blanket. The bag will turn with you and prevent cold air spaces. The bag's zipper will be easier to manipulate if it has a parachute cord "pull" attached.

Use a sleeping bag, cozy-wrap, or comforter when reading in a chair.

Use a mug to drink hot tea or coffee and hold it between both hands to warm them.

Slipper socks, worn over a pair of regular socks, will help to keep feet and ankles warm.

A foot bath not only will warm your feet as they soak in the water but also can act as a massager.

Dress warmly. Use long underwear even in the spring and fall.

Consider putting on silk or olefin long underwear under your clothes to keep warm, along with a wool sweater. This may reduce the need for heavy jackets and keep you insulated and warm.

Comfort

When sitting for long periods is necessary, such as when riding in a car or flying, you can relax your back muscles by doing the following: Place your forearms on your thighs, hands near the knees, and lean forward with your face as near to the knees as possible. Breathe deeply and relax in this position. Come up to sitting slowly; bring your head up last. Repeat several times.

Purchase a padded toilet seat or sew a toilet seat cover out of thick furry material.

Pad chairs with pillows or foam cushions.

Consider an inflatable pillow or towel rolls to make your back or neck more comfortable. Some people keep an assortment in their trunk.

If you don't want to take a pillow with you when you go out, take a sweater or jacket along to use as a cushion for hard chairs.

Recliner chairs with head supports are comfortable for many people, especially those with neck problems.

Electric beds are no longer confined to the hospital. Home models are available that have movable back and foot sections.

Be sure that you have adequate lighting and ventilation for all activities.

If you take aspirin for pain, you may want to wake up early, take your aspirin, and go back to sleep until it begins to work. Keep aspirin, crackers, and a glass of water at the bedside.

Hand, finger, thumb, and wrist splints can help to maintain joints in proper alignment and reduce stress on joints. Their most consistent impact is reduction of pain. Some people wear splints on painful wrists or painful thumbs and succeed in decreasing their pain and improving their strength during otherwise difficult activities such as cooking or using scissors. People with rheumatoid arthritis who notice alignment changes in their fingers may benefit from silver ring splints. These splints, made of silver or gold, look like jewelry and improve finger alignment. They are usually custom fit by an occupational therapist with a kit from the company. Your physician can refer you to an occupational therapist who can recommend appropriate splints for you. Splints can be custom made from hard plastic, prefabricated from soft materials or designed from silver or gold.

Knee braces often reduce knee pain. Your physician can refer you to a physical therapist to help you select the appropriate brace.

An elastic bandage (Ace) can also provide some added stability to joints, as well as serve as a reminder to use them appropriately.

A bag of frozen peas or a cold pack may feel better than heat on hot and swollen joints. Use for a maximum of twenty minutes at one time and then refrain from activity for fifteen minutes after. Do not place the cold source directly on your skin.

Miscellaneous

To control lamps, equipment, and appliances in inaccessible locations, there is a plug on the market with an on-off switch. This can be plugged in directly to a wall outlet or can be attached to an extension cord that can be positioned near you.

An easier, though more expensive, method of controlling appliances and lights is with a Home Control System. Available at stores such as Radio Shack, this device consists of a command console and up to sixteen module units for appliances. Pushing the buttons on the console will turn any appliance on or off anywhere in your house.

Use a clipboard to keep writing paper steady.

A felt-tip pen allows you to write with less pressure.

Mechanical reachers extend your reach by two to three feet (60 to 90 cm), allowing you to retrieve items from the floor or high shelves.

When attending lectures, use a cassette recorder to eliminate hurried note taking.

When shaking hands with another person, grasp the fingers or wrist of the person's hand first so that his or her thumb cannot grasp and squeeze your hand too hard.

Use a steak or paring knife at dinner because the sharper the knife, the less pressure is needed. Be careful.

Make sure the chairs you use at home are easy to get out of; if they're not, you may not want to get out of them often enough to move around and loosen up. Avoid soft, low chairs.

Identifying Resources for Support, Information, and Adaptive Equipment "Online"

Today the internet has brought to our fingertips resources that would have been extremely challenging to find just five or ten years ago. A "Google Search" can identify so many resources that it can be overwhelming to determine what you need. To ease this, a few resources are included at the end of this chapter to help you find equipment and services. They are by no means exhaustive. Each offers valuable information that you may not have found on your own. In the process of searching, you may come across other websites. Remember that all websites are not created equally. Medline Plus offers a number of resources to help you evaluate health information and web resources (www.medlineplus.com). One example is the Medline Guide to Healthy Web Surfing, www.nlm.nih.gov/medlineplus/healthywebsurfing.html.

Purchasing "Adaptive Equipment" from Catalogues and Online

Today a number of companies specialize in equipment for people with physical limitations. Pages 94–96 contain a list of companies that sell such equipment through mail-order catalogues and online. When you are choosing equipment for yourself, be selective. Identify specific tasks that interfere with your independence on a regular basis and look for equipment that is likely to make these tasks easier. For example, if opening your front door or starting your car causes hand pain, a key extender might reduce your pain. On the other hand, if holding your silverware is difficult for you, consider building up the handles with pipe-insulation tubing or buying utensils with broader handles in your local department or discount stores before shopping in catalogues. Adaptive equipment can make tasks easier and even pain-free. Sometimes using homemade adaptive equipment or modifying the way you do the activity can achieve the same goal.

Sources for Equipment

Many items described in chapters 7 and 8 are available in local department stores, hardware stores, gardening shops, or discount chain stores. You can also consider making your own adaptive aids with inexpensive supplies. Should you decide to purchase adaptive aids, some are available at medical supply stores in your area or from the companies listed below, which sell to the general public through the mail. This list is not exhaustive. If these companies here don't have what you need, seek others.

Addresses and phone numbers are included whenever available in addition to websites to accommodate those with and without a computer. A reference librarian at your local or regional library can help you locate these and other web resources. You can also use a computer yourself at your local library if you have the knowledge but not the finances to own a machine.

Selected Useful Resources

Gardening Supplies and Resources

Gardeners Supply Company
128 Intervale Road
Burlington, VT 05401
Phone: 802-660-3505, 800-955-3370
Fax: 800-551-6712
Email: info@gardeners.com
Website: www.gardeners.com

Gardens for Everybody
University of Missouri
211 Agricultural Engineering Building
Columbia, MO 65211
Phone: 573-882-2731, 800-995-8503
Website: www.fse.missouri.edu/GardenWeb/
The home page contains a picture with numbered head-
ings. Click on what interests you (e.g., special considera-
tions or ergonomic tools) and tour the breadth of
information available.

Walt Nicke Company
36 McLeod Lane
P.O. Box 433
Topsfield, MA 01983
Phone: 978-887-3388, 800-822-4114
Fax: 978-887-9853
Website: www.Gardentalk.com

Special Equipment

Freshette
The freshette system is available from Sammons Preston
Rolyan (page 96).

Intracell Stick
RPI of Atlanta
120 Interstate North Parkway East, Suite 424
Atlanta, GA 30339-2158

Phone: 770-850-1126, 800-554-1501
Fax: 770-952-7492
Email: stickdoc@intracel.net
Website: www.intracell.net

Silver Ring Splint Company
P.O. Box 2856
Charlottesville, VA 22902-2856
Phone: 800-311-7028
Fax: 888-456-8828
Email: cindy@silverringsplint.com
Website: www.silverringsplint.com

Daily Living Equipment
Hand Helpers
P.O. Box 324
Center Valley, PA 18034
Phone: 610-282-0111, 888-632-7091
Website: www.handhelpers.com

North Coast Medical, Inc.
18305 Sutter Boulevard
Morgan Hill, CA 95037-2845
Phone: 408-776-5000, 800-235-7054
Fax: 877-213-9300
Functional Solutions: home adaptive equipment
Website: www.beabletodo.com
Workplace Ergonomics: office adaptive equipment
Website: www.besafeatwork.com

Living Better with Arthritis
Aids for Arthritis, Inc.
35 Wakefield Drive
Medford, NJ 08055
Phone: 800-654-0707
Fax: 609-654-8631

Sammons Preston Rolyan
An Ability One Company
P.O. Box 5071
Bolingbrook, IL 60440-3593
Phone: 630-226-1300, 800-323-5547
Fax: 630-226-1388, 800-547-4333
Email: spr@abilityone.com
Website: www.sammonspreston.com

Arthritis Foundation
P.O. Box 7669
Atlanta, GA 30357-0669
Phone: 800-283-7800
Website: www.arthritis.org
List of easy-to-use products

Resources for Parents

Parent Empowerment Network
Website: www.disabledparents.net

Through the Looking Glass
2198 Sixth Street, Suite 100
Berkeley, CA 94710-2204
Phone: 800-644-2666 (voice)
TTY: 800-804-1616
Local: 510-848-1112
Fax: 510-848-4445
Email: TLG@lookingglass.org
Website: www.lookingglass.org

Part IV

Keeping Your Body Healthy

Chapter 9

Exercise for Fitness and Better Living

The spirit of exercise and fitness is everywhere. Well, almost everywhere. It's easy to see why arthritis and an active life can be hard to combine. When you want to exercise but aren't sure what to do, arthritis pain, stiffness, and the fear of doing harm can be powerful forces to overcome. Until recently, many people with arthritis knew they should "exercise for arthritis"; however, they thought exercising for fun and fitness was only for others.

New information has changed how we think about exercise and arthritis. Thanks to many people with arthritis who have volunteered to exercise in research studies, we can now advise exercise for fun and fitness for people with arthritis. A regular exercise program that includes flexibility, strengthening, and aerobic exercises lessens fatigue, builds stronger muscles and bones, increases your flexibility, gives you more stamina, and improves your general health and sense of well-being—all important for good arthritis care. People with arthritis have improved fitness with exercise that includes walking, bicycling, or aquatic exercise. After two or three months, most exercisers also reported less pain, anxiety, and depression.

Traditional medical care of arthritis is based on helping people mainly when their arthritis flares. During a flare, it's important to rest more and to protect the inflamed joints. But continuing to be inactive after the flare is over can be bad for your health and actually increase some arthritis problems. Unused joints, bones, and muscles deteriorate quickly. Even for someone who does not have arthritis, long periods of inactivity can lead to weakness, stiffness, fatigue, poor appetite, constipation, high blood pressure, obesity, osteoporosis, and increased sensitivity to pain, anxiety, and depression. These are some of the same problems that occur when a person has arthritis. So it can become difficult to tell whether it is arthritis, inactivity, or some combination of the two that is to blame.

In this chapter, you will learn about physical fitness and the different types of fitness exercises so you can make wise exercise choices to achieve your goals, live better and more comfortably, and be more physically fit. This advice is not intended to take the place of therapeutic exercises. If you've had an exercise plan prescribed for you or have any questions, take this book to your doctor or therapist and ask what he or she thinks about this program.

What Is Physical Fitness?

Physical fitness for people is much like good maintenance and proper use for an automobile. Both allow you to start when you want, enjoy a smooth and relaxed trip, get to your destination without a breakdown, and have some fuel in your tank when you arrive. How well an automobile works depends on its points and plugs, filters, hoses, tires, lubrication, and fuel systems.

Your physical fitness is important in determining how easy and comfortable it is for you to do what you want and need to do every day. The President's Council on Physical Fitness and Sport says, "Physical fitness is the ability to carry out daily tasks with vigor and alertness, without undue fatigue and with ample energy to engage in leisure time pursuits and to meet the above-average physical stresses of emergency situations." This is a good definition to keep in mind because it reminds us that exercise and fitness are not just for athletes and to play sports, but are important for all of us to make our lives better and more enjoyable. Physical fitness for humans is a combination of the following:

▼ Cardiovascular fitness (heart, lungs, and blood vessels)

▼ Muscle strength

▼ Muscle endurance

▼ Flexibility

▼ Percent of body fat

A regular exercise program that includes flexibility, strengthening, and aerobic activities will improve and maintain physical fitness.

Fitness is possible for people of all abilities, sizes, shapes, ages, and attitudes. Just as looking at a parked automobile doesn't tell you much about how it is driven, appearance won't tell you much about a person's physical fitness. That new, shiny model may not perform as well as the well-maintained car that has a few dents or a little rust. There is another important similarity between keeping your body fit and your car running: Both work best when used regularly and responsibly.

Regular exercise benefits everyone. By exercising, you can reduce your risk for diabetes, cardiovascular disease, and osteoporosis. You increase your stamina and have more energy. Daily tasks become easier and more comfortable. Regular exercise helps control weight and avoid constipation. When you exercise, you feel better about yourself and your abilities.

Physical Fitness and Arthritis

People who are physically active are healthier, happier, more productive, and live longer than people who are sedentary. This is true for everyone, including people with arthritis. However, arthritis is one of the most common reasons people give up or limit physical activities. We now know that inactivity causes weakness, stiffness, increased pain, poor endurance, fatigue, and other problems that we used to blame on arthritis.

If you have arthritis, regular exercise and fitness have special benefits above and beyond the general benefits of improved health.

1. Strong muscles that do not tire quickly help protect joints by improving stability and absorbing shock.

2. Good flexibility lessens pain and reduces the risk of sprains and strains.

3. Maintaining a good weight helps take stress off weight-bearing joints.

4. Regular exercise that moves the joints improves joint circulation and nutrition, decreases joint swelling, and keeps cartilage and bone healthy.

5. Regular exercise and fitness also result in higher energy levels, less depression and pain, better balance, and greater comfort doing daily activities.

Thinking of your exercise as a physical fitness program helps you take a positive, mainstream approach to exercise. By understanding physical fitness and exercise, you'll be able to improve your health, feel better, and manage your arthritis, too. Feeling more in control and less at the mercy of arthritis is one of the greatest benefits of becoming an exercise self-manager.

Your Own Fitness Program

An exercise program to improve physical fitness includes exercises for flexibility, strength, endurance, and cardiovascular fitness. How you choose to combine these different types of exercise depends on your current abilities, exercise experience, and the goals you want to accomplish.

To be a successful exercise self-manager, you need to understand what the different types of exercise can do for you and how to use them to meet your goals. The following section introduces you to the three basic types of exercise: flexibility, strengthening, and aerobic exercise. The Fitness Exercises table on page 103 is a quick exercise reference. Details and instructions for doing the exercises are in chapters 10, 11, and 12.

Flexibility Exercises

Flexibility exercises, also known as range-of-motion and stretching exercises, are the foundation of any exercise program. They are especially important for the person with arthritis. The purpose is to increase or maintain flexibility and motion in muscles, tendons, ligaments, and joints. Flexibility is necessary for comfortable movement during exercise and daily activities and to reduce the risk of sprains and strains. Flexibility is also important for good posture, strength, and balance.

Flexibility exercises are done gently and smoothly, three to ten times each, usually every day. Flexibility exercises should also be performed before any more vigorous type of exercise and can be good warm-ups for daily tasks.

If you haven't exercised regularly in some time or have pain, stiffness, or weakness that interferes with your daily activities, begin your fitness program by building a routine of fifteen minutes of the flexibility exercises. When you can do fifteen minutes of continuous flexibil-

Fitness Exercises: Quick-Reference Guide

Type	Suggestions for use	Benefits
Flexibility	Daily routine; get in shape for strengthening/aerobics; aerobics warm-up; as needed for comfort; warm-up or cool-down for daily activities	Flexibility; comfort; joint health; easier daily activity; relaxation
Strength	Every-other-day routine; with flexibility exercise; with flexibility and aerobic for total fitness program; combine upper- and lower-body exercises	Protect joints; easier daily activity; relieve pain; reduce fatigue; strengthen bones; increase endurance
Aerobic	Every-other-day routine; short bouts several times a day; alternate brisk exercise with slow exercise to build up total duration of aerobic activity	General health; increase energy; weight control; improve mood; sleep better; increase stamina; lower blood pressure; strengthen bones; relaxation

ity exercise, you will have the motion and endurance needed to include strengthening and aerobic exercise in your fitness program. Flexibility exercises are shown and described in Chapter 10.

Strengthening Exercises

Strengthening exercises, sometimes called resistance exercises, are important for everyone, especially for a person with arthritis. Joint swelling and pain can make muscles weak. Not using muscles because of stiffness and pain can also lead to weakness. Weak muscles are a special problem if you have arthritis because strong muscles help absorb shock, support joints, and protect you from injuries. Strong muscles also improve balance, endurance, and the ability to safely walk, climb stairs, lift, and reach. Strengthening exercises are part of your fitness program and of good arthritis self-management.

Strengthening exercises ask your muscles to work a little harder than usual. When you ask your muscles to do a little more on a regular basis, your muscles gradually adapt to the extra work by getting stronger. Strengthening exercises add resistance (extra work) by using the weight of your body, extra weights you hold, or elastic bands. The secret of a good strengthening program is to "overload" your muscles just enough to get them to adapt but not so much that they are sore and stiff a day or two after you exercised.

If you have particular joint problems or have been told to protect certain joints, check with a therapist about what strengthening exercises are best and safest for you. If you have not been active in some time, it is best to build up to fifteen minutes of flexibility exercises before adding strengthening to your program. Strengthening exercises are shown and explained in Chapter 11.

Aerobic Exercises

Many people think that aerobic exercise is not for them. When they hear the word *aerobic,* they think of people in crazy clothes jumping around to loud music. It is important to understand that aerobic exercise does not mean just "aerobic dance." Aerobic exercise, also known as endurance or cardiovascular exercise, is any physical activity that uses the large muscles of your body in rhythmic, continuous motions. The most effective types of aerobic exercise use your whole body: walking, dancing, swimming, bicycling, mowing the lawn, or even raking leaves.

The purpose of aerobic exercise is to improve the ability of your heart, lungs, blood vessels, and muscles to work efficiently and effectively. You can do this by asking your body to do just a bit more aerobic exercise than it does now. Your body will adapt to a regular program of aerobic exercise by becoming more "aerobically fit."

When you are aerobically fit, your heart doesn't have to beat so fast and it can pump more blood out to your body with each beat. Your blood vessels can carry enough blood to deliver oxygen to all parts of your body, and your muscles can work longer and harder with less fatigue. You are at less risk for problems such as heart disease, high blood pressure, and diabetes. Aerobic exercise is the kind of exercise that helps control weight, improve sleep, strengthen bones, reduce depression and anxiety, and build endurance. Aerobic exercise is really quite a bargain when you think of all the benefits you can gain.

A fitness program needs to include some aerobic activities three to four days a week. Chapter 12 explains ways for you to include aerobic exercise in your fitness program and gives guidelines for deciding how much to do and how hard to work.

How Much Exercise Is Enough?

How often you exercise, what you do, and how much you do depend on your health and fitness now and what you want to accomplish with exercise. When it comes to exercise, remember that more is not always better. It is important to know when you have reached your goal and can say, "This is right for me." Chapters 10, 11, and 12 will give you more information about exercise frequency, intensity, and duration. For now, you can see from the recommendations below that being able to exercise and be active for better health or fitness is a real possibility for everyone.

How much exercise is enough for general health? To be active enough to be in the category of people who have less risk of heart disease, diabetes, and high blood pressure than people who are sedentary and do no physical activity, follow these guidelines from the U.S. Surgeon General's *Report on Physical Activity and Health*.

If setting aside a special time to just exercise is not something you think you are going to do, try increasing your active time by adding more physical activity to what you do every day. For example, park the car a little farther away from the door, do something that requires getting up and walking a short distance every hour, walk the dog a little longer.

Physical Activity Recommendation for Health

Type of activity: Aerobic activities such as walking or biking; or regular daily activities such as sweeping, raking leaves, making beds, mowing the lawn, or washing the car

Frequency: On most days of the week

Intensity: Low to moderate exertion

Duration: Accumulate at least 30 minutes each day (the goal can be to work up to 10 minutes 3 times a day)

To increase your all-around fitness and see improvements in your flexibility, strength, endurance, and weight, you will need to gradually build your exercise program until you can follow these guidelines:

Exercise Recommendation for Fitness

Types of exercise: Flexibility, strengthening, aerobic

Frequency: Flexibility—3 to 7 days a week
Strengthening—2 to 3 days a week
Aerobic—3 to 4 days a week

Intensity: Strengthening—Low to moderate exertion
Aerobic—Moderate intensity

Duration: Strengthening—10 repetitions of 8 to 10
exercises
Aerobic—30 to 40 minutes

Preparing to Exercise

Figuring out how to make the commitment of time and energy to regular exercise is a challenge for everyone. If you have arthritis, you have even more challenges. You must take precautions and find a program that is safe and comfortable. You also have to understand how to adapt your exercise to changes in your arthritis and joint problems. Learning how much is enough before you've done too much is especially important.

Start by learning your arthritis needs. If possible, talk with your doctor and other professionals who understand your kind of arthritis. Get their ideas about special exercise needs and precautions. Read the section "Exercise Ideas for Specific Diseases" at the end of this chapter (page 113). Learn to be aware of your own body, and plan your activities accordingly. Your personal exercise program should be based on *your* current level of health and fitness, *your* goals and desires, *your* abilities and special needs, and *your* likes and dislikes. Deciding to improve your fitness, and feeling the satisfaction of success, has nothing to do with competition or comparing yourself to others.

Opportunities in Your Community

Most people who exercise regularly do so with at least one other person. Two or more people can keep each other motivated, and a whole class can build a feeling of camaraderie. On the other hand, exercising alone gives you the most freedom. You may feel that there are no classes that would work for you or no buddy to exercise with. If so, start your own program. As you progress, you may find that these feelings change.

The Arthritis Foundation, Arthritis Society, and Arthritis Care sponsor exercise programs taught by trained instructors and developed specifically for people with arthritis. Consult your local chapter or branch office.

Most communities now offer a variety of exercise classes, including special programs for people over fifty, adaptive exercises, mall walking, fitness trails, and others. Check with the local Y, community and senior centers, parks and recreation programs, adult education, and community colleges. Many hospitals sponsor employee and community fitness and health promotion programs. There is a great deal of variation in the content of these programs, as well as in the professional experience of the exercise staff. By and large, the classes are inexpensive, and those in charge of planning are responsive to people's needs.

Health and fitness clubs usually offer aerobic studios, weight training, cardiovascular equipment, and sometimes a heated pool. For all these services they charge membership and class fees. Make sure you understand the financial commitment before you sign up. Ask about low-impact, beginners, and over-fifty exercise classes, both in the aerobic studio and in the pool. Gyms that emphasize weight lifting generally don't have the programs or personnel to help you with a flexible, all-around fitness program. These are some qualities you should look for in a health club:

▼ **Classes** that are designed for moderate- and low-intensity exercise. You should be able to observe classes and participate in at least one class before committing.

▼ **Instructors** who have qualifications and experience. Knowledgeable instructors are more likely to understand special needs and be willing and able to work with you.

▼ **Membership policies** that allow you to pay only for a session of classes, or let you "freeze" membership at times when you can't participate. Some fitness facilities offer different rates depending on how many services you use. Some use a "punch card" system that gives you lots of flexibility.

▼ **Facilities** that are easy to get to, park near, and enter. Dressing rooms and exercise sites should be accessible and safe, with professional staff on-site.

▼ A **pool** that allows "free swim" times when the water isn't crowded. Also, find out the policy about children in the pool; small children playing and making noise may not be compatible with your needs.

▼ **Staff and other members** with whom you feel comfortable.

Putting Your Program Together

The best way to enjoy and stick with your exercise program is to suit yourself! Choose what you want to do, a place where you feel comfortable, and an exercise time that fits your schedule. A young mother with school-age children will find it difficult to stick with an exercise program that requires her to leave home for a five o'clock class. A retired man who enjoys lunch with friends and an afternoon nap is wise to choose an early- or mid-morning exercise time.

Having fun and enjoying yourself are benefits of exercise that often go unmentioned. Too often we think of exercise as serious business. However, most people who stick with a program do so because they enjoy it. They think of their exercise as recreation rather than a chore. Start off with success in mind. Allow yourself time to get used to new experiences, and you'll probably find that you look forward to exercise.

Some well-meaning health professionals can make it hard for a person with arthritis to stick to an exercise program. You may have been prescribed exercises to do on your own at home (sometimes four times a day) for the rest of your life! What a lonely-sounding chore! No wonder so many people never start or give up quickly. Not many of us make lifelong commitments to unknown projects. Experience, practice, and success are necessary to establish a habit. Follow the self-management steps in Chapter 6 to make beginning your program easier.

Having an exercise goal, making an exercise plan to achieve that goal, and keeping track of progress are important parts of a satisfying and successful exercise program.

Ensuring Your Exercise Success

1. **Select a problem you would like to solve or a goal you would like to achieve.** Pick something that you want to do that is related to your physical abilities, such as being able to walk on the beach during vacation, get in and out of the tub, spend a day shopping with friends, or walk your dog.

2. **Explore reasons why you can't or don't do it now.** Think about what you could change about your physical fitness (strength, flexibility, endurance, weight) that would be helpful. For example, a man who wanted to be able to get in and out of his deep bathtub by himself decided that he needed to be able to bend his knees farther and have stronger leg and shoulder muscles. A woman whose goal was to

walk on the beach decided she needed more flexibility and strength in her ankles and better general endurance.

3. **Choose exercises that can solve the problems you have identified.** Combine any prescribed exercises with exercises from the next three chapters. Talk with other people with arthritis who exercise to get more ideas about helpful exercises.

4. **Make an Exercise Action Plan.** Your action plan states your goal and includes your chosen exercises, the time and place to exercise, and how long you will stick with this plan. Six to twelve weeks is a reasonable time commitment for a new program. Share your action plan with your family and friends. (See Chapter 6, "Becoming an Arthritis Self-Manager," for more ideas about filling out your action plan.)

5. **Do some self-tests.** You will find these at the end of each of the next three chapters. Record the results and dates on your Fitness Record.

6. **Start your program.** Remember to begin gradually and be realistic with your expectations if you haven't exercised in a while.

7. **Keep a Fitness Record or Exercise Calendar.** This may be as simple as check marks on a calendar or keeping a journal in which you record what you did and how you felt. Keep your record where you can see it and fill it out every day.

8. **Keep an eye on your goal and repeat the self-tests.** After about four weeks, see if you are making progress toward your goal; repeat the self-tests and record your findings. You can repeat self-tests every three to four weeks or choose new self-tests to check progress.

9. **Check your results and make your next plan.** At the end of the time period you chose, assess the results. Decide if you have made progress, what you liked, what worked, and what didn't. Modify your exercise action plan and try the new plan for another few weeks. You may decide to change what you are doing, when or where you exercise, or your exercise partners. This may be a time to update your goal.

10. **Reward yourself for a job well done.** Make sure you take the time to enjoy your successes and congratulate yourself.

Keeping It Up

If you haven't exercised recently, you'll undoubtedly experience some new feelings and discomfort in the early days. It's normal to feel muscle tension and possibly tenderness around joints, and to be a little more tired in the evenings. Muscle or joint pain that lasts more than two hours after the exercise or feeling tired into the next day means that you probably did too much too fast. Don't stop; just exercise less vigorously or for a shorter time the next day.

When you do aerobic exercise, it's natural to feel your heart beat faster, your breathing speed up, and your body get warmer. Feeling short of breath, nauseated, or dizzy, however, is not what you want. If this happens to you, stop exercising and discontinue your program until you check with your doctor.

People who have arthritis have additional sensations to sort out. It can be difficult at first to figure out which sensations come from arthritis and which come from exercise. Talking to someone else with arthritis who has had experience starting a new exercise program can be a big help. Once you've sorted out the new sensations, you'll be able to exercise with confidence.

Think of your head as the coach and your body as your team. For success, all parts of the team need attention. Be a good coach. Encourage and praise yourself. Design "plays" you feel your team can execute successfully. Choose places that are safe and hospitable. A good coach knows his or her team, sets good goals, and helps the team succeed. A good coach is loyal. A good coach does not belittle, nag, or make anyone feel guilty. Be a good coach to your team.

Besides a good coach, everyone needs an enthusiastic cheerleader or two. Of course, you can be your own cheerleader, but being both coach and cheerleader is a lot to do. Successful exercisers usually have at least one family member or close friend who actively supports their exercise habit. Your cheerleader can exercise with you, help you get other chores done, praise your accomplishments, or just consider your exercise time when making plans. Sometimes cheerleaders pop up by themselves, but don't be bashful about asking for a hand.

With exercise experience, you develop a sense of control over yourself and your arthritis. You learn how to alternate your activities to fit your day-to-day needs. You know when to do less and when to do more. You know that a flare, or a period of inactivity in taking care of the arthritis, doesn't have to be devastating. You know how to get back on track again.

Give your exercise plan a chance to succeed. Set reasonable goals and enjoy your success. Stay motivated. When it comes to your personal fitness program, sticking with it and doing it your way make you a definite winner.

Exercise Ideas for Specific Diseases

Everything we've suggested up to now applies to everyone with arthritis. Here are some additional exercise ideas and tips for people with specific diseases.

Osteoarthritis

Since osteoarthritis is primarily a problem with joint cartilage, an exercise program should include taking care of cartilage. Cartilage needs joint motion to stay healthy. In much the same way that a sponge soaks up and squeezes out water, joint cartilage soaks up nutrients and fluid and gets rid of waste products by being squeezed when you move the joint. If the joint is not moved regularly, cartilage deteriorates. If the joint is continually compressed, as the hips and knees are by long periods of standing, the cartilage can't expand and soak up nutrients and fluid.

Any joint with osteoarthritis should be moved through its full range of motion several times daily to maintain flexibility and to take care of the cartilage. Judge your activity level so that pain is not increased. If hips and knees are involved, walking and standing should be limited to no more than two to four hours at a time, followed by at least an hour off your feet to give cartilage time to decompress. If you have knee osteoarthritis, knee-strengthening exercises (see pages 156–159) can decrease your knee pain and make it easier and more comfortable for you to walk, get up and down from a chair, and climb stairs. Good posture, strong muscles with good endurance, and shoes that absorb the shocks of walking are important ways to protect cartilage and reduce joint pain.

Rheumatoid Arthritis

People with rheumatoid arthritis should pay special attention to flexibility, strengthening, and appropriate use of their joints. Maintaining good posture and joint motion will help joints, ease pain, and avoid tightness. Arthritis pain and long periods spent sitting or lying down can quickly lead to poor posture and limited motion, even in the joints not affected by the arthritis. Be sure to include hand and wrist exercises in your daily program (see pages 129–131). A good time to do these is after washing dishes or during a bath when hands are warm and more limber.

Rheumatoid arthritis sometimes affects the bones in the neck. It is best to avoid extreme neck movements and not to put pressure on the back of the neck or head.

Stiffness in the morning can be a big problem. Flexibility exercises before getting up or during a hot bath or shower seem to help. A favorite way to get loosened up is to "stretch like a cat." Also, doing gentle flexibility exercises in the evening before bed can help reduce morning stiffness.

Ankylosing Spondylitis and Psoriatic Arthritis

Ankylosing spondylitis and psoriatic arthritis can result in loss of motion in the neck, back, and hips. Flexibility exercises, especially for the neck, spine, shoulders, and hips, are important parts of the exercise program, along with breathing and chest expansion. Muscle-strengthening exercises for back and hips are also needed to maintain erect posture. Correct head and neck posture is also extremely important to maintain good alignment and reduce pain with activity.

In these diseases, inflammation of muscles, tendons, and ligaments also occurs, making them vulnerable to injuries and sprains. Repeated inflammation can result in shortening and thickening of tissue around joints and lead to loss of motion. Therefore, it is extremely important to do regular flexibility exercises. Exercise gently, with slow, controlled movements and held positions. Bouncing or jerking is dangerous.

The Achilles tendon or heel cord is especially at risk. Use the Achilles Stretch (page 143) to keep the heel cord and tissue covering the sole of the foot elastic. This helps reduce the chance of tendon tears, plantar fasciitis, heel pain, and heel spurs. Resting for some time each day on your stomach with your feet hanging over the end of the bed is another way to encourage good posture.

Stiffness in the neck and spine doesn't mean you can't be physically fit. Swimming is an excellent exercise. Swimming strengthens back, shoulders, and hips and provides a good cardiovascular workout. Use a snorkel and mask to allow you to swim without turning your head to breathe.

Systemic Lupus Erythematosus (SLE)

The fatigue and joint pains that so many people with SLE experience can be a major stumbling block to being active. These problems can be improved with a regular program of moderate exercise undertaken when the disease process is under control. A program that includes flexibility, strengthening, and aerobic exercise is appropriate. It is wise to avoid high-impact activities such as jumping or bouncing, especially if you're taking oral corticosteroids. If you start to have pain in your hip or groin, check with your doctor to make sure you are not having hip problems. Combining walking, bicycling, and swimming or pool exercise will give you a well-balanced program with maximum safety. Nighttime flexibility exercises may help reduce morning stiffness.

Raynaud's Phenomenon

If cold sensitivity or Raynaud's phenomenon is a problem, avoid extreme temperature changes when you plan your exercise. If you live where there are cold winters, develop a good indoor exercise program. Some people have found that wearing disposable latex surgical gloves underneath a pair of regular gloves or mittens is useful. If you like water exercise but the water temperature is too cold for your hands, try putting on latex gloves before getting in the water.

Osteoporosis

Regular exercise at all ages plays an important part in preventing osteoporosis and in strengthening bones that already show signs of the disease. Endurance exercises such as walking are effective for strengthening bone. Strengthening exercises for back and stomach muscles are necessary for maintaining good posture and also help strengthen the spine. The exercises marked VIP (very important for posture) and upper-body-strengthening exercises (see pages 160–164) are particularly useful.

You can help yourself with a regular exercise program that includes some walking and general flexibility and strengthening of your back, shoulders, hips, and stomach muscles.

If you have osteoporosis or think you may be at risk for this condition, here are some exercise precautions for you to remember:

▼ No heavy lifting.

▼ Avoid falls. Be careful on pool decks, waxed floors, icy sidewalks, or cluttered surfaces.

▼ Don't bend down to touch your toes when standing. This puts unnecessary pressure on your back. If you want to stretch your legs or back, lie on your back and bring your knees up toward your chest.

▼ Sit up straight and don't slouch. Good sitting posture puts less pressure on the back.

▼ If your balance is poor or you feel clumsy, consider using a cane or walking stick when you're in a crowd or on unfamiliar ground.

Fibromyalgia
This condition can occur by itself or appear in people who also have other forms of arthritis. The symptoms are stiffness, fatigue, general aching, and extremely tender spots around the shoulders, upper back, hips, and knees. There are no signs of inflammation or joint involvement (see Chapter 5). Exercise for this condition is very useful. It seems that a very slow increase in

aerobic activity is the most important aspect of treatment in fibromyalgia. Exercises to develop good posture, flexibility, and gentle strengthening can also help. Low to moderate aerobic exercise, such as walking, should be slowly progressed toward thirty minutes a day, and then the intensity increased. People with fibromyalgia often get worse after doing very vigorous exercise for which they have not trained. Exercise can help reduce muscle tension, decrease pain, aid relaxation, and improve sleep. Exercise is an important treatment for fibromyalgia.

Chapter 10
Flexibility Exercises

This chapter illustrates and explains flexibility exercises. Use these exercises to:

▼ Improve flexibility

▼ Get in shape for more vigorous exercise

▼ Keep the exercise habit on days when you don't do other kinds of exercise

▼ Warm up before and cool down after aerobic exercise

▼ Get ready for a daily activity such as yard work or shopping

▼ Stretch and relax after a tiring activity such as gardening or housekeeping

If you are not exercising regularly now or if you have pain or stiffness that interferes with your daily activities, start your program with exercises from this chapter. Gradually build up the number and repetitions to a fifteen-minute session. When you can do a continuous fifteen minutes of flexibility exercises, gradually add strengthening and aerobic exercises (see chapters 11 and 12). Choose exercises to build a program for the whole body.

Exercises are arranged in groups for different parts of the body. You can choose the positions and exercises that best suit you. Most of the upper-body exercises may be done either sitting or standing. Exercises done lying down can be performed on the floor or on a firm mattress. We've labeled the exercises that are particularly important for good posture "VIP" (very important for posture).

Tips for Flexibility Exercises

Follow these helpful hints when you do flexibility exercises:

▼ Move slowly and gently. Do not bounce or jerk.

▼ To loosen tight muscles and limber up stiff joints, stretch just until you feel tension and then hold for a count of fifteen, up to a count of thirty.

▼ Start with no more than five repetitions of any exercise. Take at least two weeks to increase to ten.

▼ Arrange your exercises so you don't have to get up and down a lot.

▼ Always do the same exercises for your left side as for your right.

▼ Breathe naturally. Do not hold your breath. Count out loud to make sure that you are breathing easily.

▼ If you have increased pain that lasts more than two hours after exercising, do fewer repetitions next time or eliminate an exercise that seems to be causing the pain. Don't stop exercising.

Neck Flexibility Exercises

1. Chin In (VIP)

This exercise relieves jaw, neck, and upper-back pain and is the start of good posture. You can do it as part of your exercise routine or while driving, sitting at a desk, sewing, or reading. Just sit or stand straight and gently slide your chin back. Keep looking forward as your chin moves backward. You'll feel the back of your neck lengthen and straighten. To help, put your finger on your nose and then draw straight back from your finger. (Don't worry about a little double chin—you really look much better with your neck straight!)

If it's uncomfortable for you to do this exercise at first, practice the movement lying flat on your back on the floor or on a firm mattress without a pillow. In this position, pull your chin in by pressing the base of your skull into the floor or mattress. As your neck becomes more flexible, you will be able to hold this good head position comfortably when you are sitting and standing.

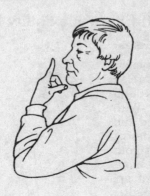

2. Two-Way Neck Stretch

Start in chin-in position (Exercise 1), and with your shoulders relaxed,

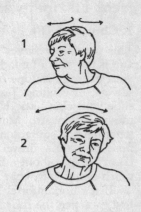

1. Turn slowly to look over your right shoulder. Then turn slowly to look over your left shoulder.

2. Tilt your head to the right and then to the left. Move your ear toward your shoulder. Do not move your shoulder up to your ear.

If these exercises make you dizzy, close your eyes. If you are still dizzy, skip it. Don't do these exercises if they cause neck pain or pain or numbness in your arms or hands.

Shoulder and Elbow Flexibility Exercises

3. Shoulder Circles

You can do this exercise anytime to relax your shoulders and upper back. With shoulders relaxed and arms at your sides or hands resting in your lap, gently roll your shoulders forward, up, back, and down. Reverse and go the other way.

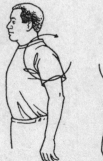
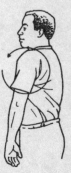

4. Sunrise Stretch (VIP)

You can do this stretch either sitting or standing.

1. Relax your arms, cross your wrists in front of you, and make gentle fists with your thumbs pointing down.

2. Start the movement with your hands. Roll your hands over, straighten fingers, move your arms upward and outward, and reach as high up as you can. Breathe in as you raise your arms.

3. Relax and return to the starting position, and breathe out as you bring your arms down.

   This exercise encourages good posture and is a relaxing stretch for your upper body.

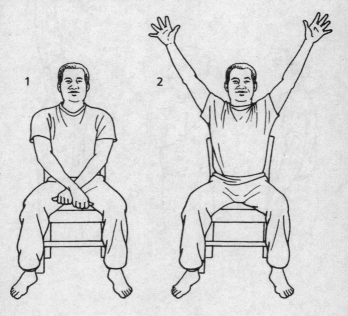

5. Bend and Reach

You can sit, stand, or lie on your back to do this exercise.

1. Start with your arms relaxed and elbows straight.

2. Bend your elbows to bring your hands up to touch your shoulders.

3. Then reach your hands up to the ceiling as you straighten your elbows. Reach as high as you can, stretching elbows and shoulders.

4. Breathe in as you stretch up and breathe out as you relax back to the starting position.

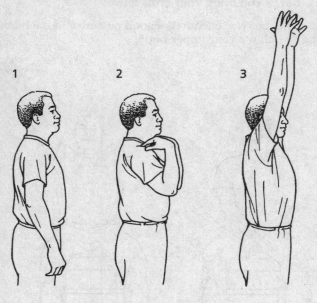

1   2   3

6. Pat and Reach

This double-duty exercise helps increase flexibility both in elbows and in shoulders.

1. Raise one arm over your head and bend your elbow to pat yourself on the back.

2. Move your other arm to your back, bend your elbow, and reach up toward the other hand. Can your fingertips touch?

3. Relax and switch arm positions. Can you touch on that side? For most people, one position will work better than the other.

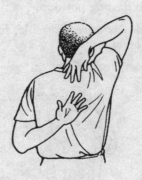

7. Shoulder Roll and Squeeze (VIP)

This is a good exercise to strengthen the middle and upper back and to stretch the chest.

1. Sit or stand with your head in chin-in position (Exercise 1) and your shoulders relaxed. Raise your arms to shoulder level out to the sides, with elbows bent and fingertips pointed down.

2. Roll your hands upward until you are in a "stick 'em up" position.

3. Pinch your shoulder blades together by moving your elbows as far back as you can. Hold briefly. Relax and return to starting position.

   If this exercise is uncomfortable, lower your arms below shoulder level.

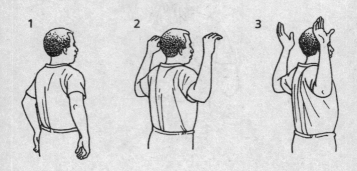

8. Shoulder Pulley

Fasten a hook or pulley in a beam or on the top of a door frame. Place a piece of rope or clothesline through the hook, as shown. Start with enough rope so you can sit while exercising. Hold one end of the rope in each hand. If gripping the rope is uncomfortable, add padding or handles. As you pull down with one arm, the other arm will be raised. Stand (or sit) so your arms clear the frame. Move your arms up and down in front of you and also out to the side.

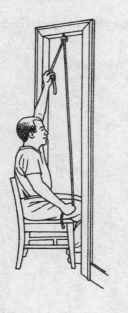
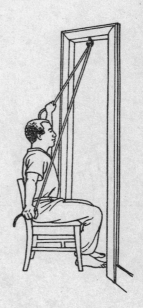

9. Wand Exercise

This shoulder exercise and the preceding one allow the arms to help each other. If one or both of your shoulders are particularly tight or weak, you may find this a "helping hand."

Use a cane, yardstick, or mop handle as your wand. Place your hands about shoulder width apart and raise the wand as high overhead as possible. You might try this in front of a mirror. This wand exercise can be done standing, sitting, or lying down.

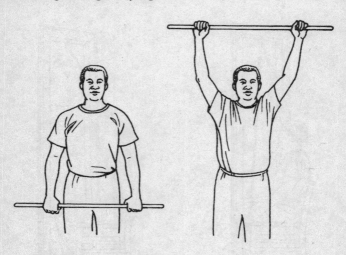

Hand and Wrist Flexibility Exercises

A good place to do these hand exercises is at a table that supports your forearms. Do them after washing dishes, after bathing, or as a break from handwork.

10. One-Two-Three Finger Exercises

For the best hand function, you should be able to make a loose fist with your thumb crossed over your fingers and also be able to straighten your fingers completely. Use the one-two-three approach.

1. Begin bending the middle finger joints, then bend your knuckles so your fingertips are as close as possible to your palm.

2. Cross your thumb over your fingers toward your little finger.

3. Hold this position momentarily and then straighten your fingers and spread them wide apart. Use one hand to help the other if necessary.

1   2   3

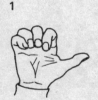 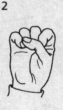 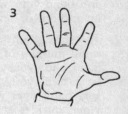

11. Thumb Walk

1. Holding your wrist straight, form the letter O by lightly touching your thumb to each fingertip.

2. After forming each O, straighten and spread your fingers. Use the other hand to help if needed.

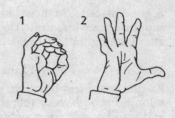

12. Hi and Bye (Hello and Cheerio)

1. To strengthen and limber your wrist, rest your forearm on a table with your hand over the edge. Keep fingers relaxed and bend your wrist up and down.

2. To strengthen the small muscles of the hand, slide your arm back until your fingers hang over with your knuckles at the table edge. Keeping your fingers straight and together and your palm flat, move your fingers up and down.

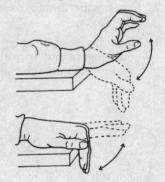

13. Door Opener

This is an exercise to stretch the muscles and ligaments that rotate the forearm, letting you turn doorknobs, use a screwdriver, or put your hand in your back pocket.

1. Start with your forearm resting on a table, palm down.

2. Keeping your upper arm and elbow tucked in close to your side and your little finger on the table, turn your hand so the palm faces up. Do not move your upper arm or elbow.

If you use your other hand to help, grip your forearm, not the wrist or hand.

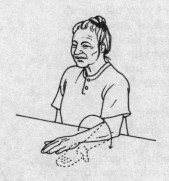

Trunk and Back Flexibility Exercises

14. Trunk Twist

You can do this stretch either sitting or standing. Move your arms to shoulder level or cross them over your chest. Slowly and gently twist at the waist to one side and then the other. Turn your head with your torso so that you don't twist your neck. Don't turn your head too far—this exercise is for your back. The purpose is to increase the flexibility of your trunk and make it easier and more comfortable for you to turn and roll. It will help loosen up your back to prepare for other exercise, such as walking or dancing.

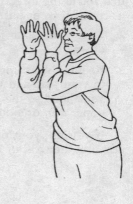

15. Up and Over

This is a good stretch for trunk, shoulders, elbows, and hands. Sitting or standing, reach one arm up over your head and then reach with that hand over toward your other side, leaning your trunk slightly in that direction. You should feel a stretch along your trunk on the reaching side. Relax. Stretch your fingers out straight when you reach up and make a loose fist as you move back down. Do the same thing on the other side.

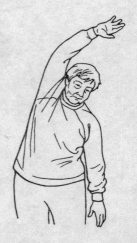

16. Pelvic Tilt (VIP)

This is an excellent exercise for lower-back pain. It can be done on the floor or on a firm mattress.

1. Lie on your back with your knees bent, feet flat. Place your hands on your abdomen.

2. Flatten the small of your back against the floor by tightening your stomach muscles and your buttocks. It helps to imagine bringing your pubic bone to your chin or trying to pull your tummy in enough to zip a tight pair of trousers.

3. Hold the tilt for five to ten seconds. Relax.

4. Arch your back slightly. Relax.

5. Repeat the Pelvic Tilt. Keep breathing. Count the seconds out loud.

Once you've mastered the Pelvic Tilt lying down, practice it sitting, standing, and walking.

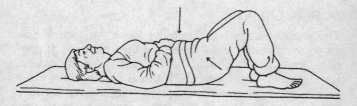

17. Lower-Back Rock and Roll

1. Lie on your back on the floor or a firm mattress and pull your knees up to your chest with your hands behind the thighs. Rest in this position for ten seconds.

2. Gently roll knees from one side to the other, rocking your hips back and forth. Keep your upper back and shoulders flat on the floor or mattress.

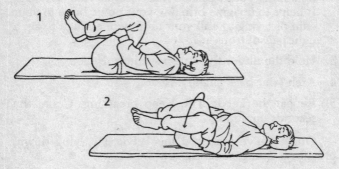

18. Back Lift (VIP)

This exercise improves flexibility along your spine. Lie on your stomach on the floor or a firm mattress. If possible, your hands should be beneath your shoulders. Rise up onto your forearms. If this is comfortable, keep your hands in place and straighten your elbows. Breathe naturally and relax. If you have moderate to severe lower-back pain, do not do this exercise unless it has been specifically prescribed for you. This is not a good exercise if you have spinal stenosis.

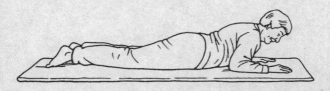

19. Knee-to-Chest Stretch

1. For a hip and lower-back stretch, lie on the floor or on a firm mattress with knees bent and feet flat.

2. Bring one knee toward your chest, using your hands to help.

3. Hold your knee near your chest for ten seconds and lower the leg slowly.

4. Repeat with the other knee.

To get more lower-back stretch, tuck both legs at the same time. Relax and enjoy the stretch.

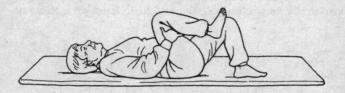

20. Cat Back and Sway

This is a good way to loosen up your back and strengthen stomach muscles, as well.

1. On hands and knees, on forearms and knees, or leaning over a counter or table, relax and let your back sway and your stomach sag.

2. Slowly arch your back like a mad cat as you tighten and pull in your stomach.

3. Relax your back and let it sway again.

4. Repeat the whole sequence.

Be sure to keep looking at the floor and to breathe naturally as you move back and forth from arch to sway.

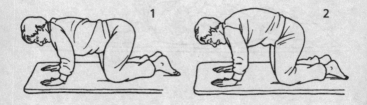

Hip and Knee Flexibility Exercises

21. Hip Rolls

This is an important exercise to keep the hip flexible and in good position for comfortable walking and standing up straight.

1. Stand with one foot slightly in front of the other. Slightly bend the hip and knee of the forward leg so that your heel is off the floor.

2. Keeping your foot in place and swiveling on your toes, roll your knee in, then out. Although you can see your knee moving, the motion is really in your hip.

If you have hip pain when you stand on one foot, you can do this movement lying down (Hip Hooray, Exercise 23).

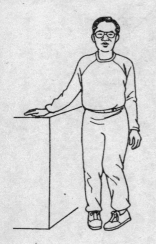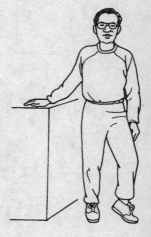

22. Back Kick (VIP)

This exercise increases the backward mobility and strength of your hip. Hold on to a counter for support. Move the leg backward and forward. Keep your knee fairly straight and do not point your toes. Stand tall and do not arch your back.

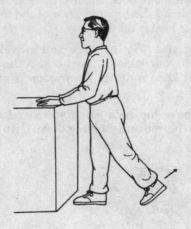

23. Hip Hooray

This exercise can be done lying on your back (A) or standing (B).

A. If you lie down, spread your legs as far apart as possible. Roll your legs and feet out like a duck and then in, pigeon-toed. Keep your knees straight.

B. If you are standing, hold on to a counter for support. Move one leg out to your side as far as you can. Roll your leg to turn your toes inward when you move your leg out; then point your toes outward as you return to the starting position.

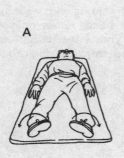

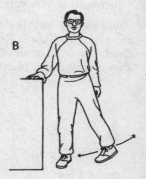

24. Hamstring Stretch

This exercise helps loosen tight hamstrings. Do the self-test for hamstring tightness (page 174) to see if you need to do this exercise. It is also a good exercise to do if you get muscle cramps in the back of your thigh. If you have unstable knees, or "back knee" (a knee that curves backward when you stand up), do not do this exercise.

A. 1. Lie on your back, knees bent, feet flat.

   2. Bend one hip so your leg is at about a right angle with the body.

   3. Slowly straighten the knee. Hold the leg as straight as you can as you count to fifteen.

B. You can also do this exercise by sitting with your foot on a low footstool. Rest your hands either on your thighs or at your sides. With your knee straight and toes pointed up, lean forward from the hips (back

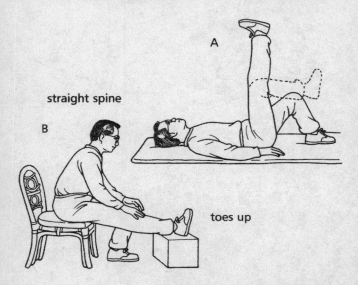

straight spine

A

B

toes up

straight) until you feel a stretch on the back of your leg. Hold and count to fifteen. Relax.

Be careful with this exercise. It's easy to overstretch and be sore.

Ankle and Foot Flexibility Exercises

Do these exercises sitting in a straight-backed chair with your feet bare. Have a bath towel and ten marbles or small paper wads next to you. These exercises are for flexibility, relaxation, and comfort.

25. Ankle Circles

With your heels on the floor, slowly circle your feet to the right and then to the left. Go as far in each direction as you can.

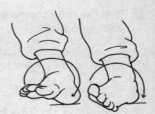

26. Towel Grabber

1. Spread a towel out in front of your chair. Place your feet on the towel with your heels on the edge closest to you. Keep your heels down.

2. Scoot the towel back underneath your feet by pulling it with your toes as you arch your feet.

3. When you have done as much as you can, reverse the toe motion and scoot the towel out again.

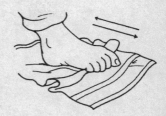

You may do both feet together or separately.

27. Marble Pickup

Do this exercise one foot at a time. Place several marbles on the floor between your feet.

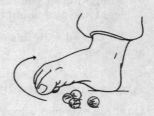

1. Keep your heel down and pivot your toes toward the marbles.

2. Pick up a marble in your toes and pivot your foot to drop the marble as far as possible from where you picked it up.

3. Repeat until all the marbles have been moved.

4. Reverse the process and return all the marbles to the starting position.

If marbles are difficult, try other objects like jacks, dice, or wads of paper.

28. Foot Roll

Place a rolling pin (or a large dowel or closet rod) under the arch of your foot and roll it back and forth. It feels great and stretches the ligaments in the arch of the foot.

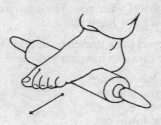

29. Achilles Stretch

This exercise helps maintain flexibility in the Achilles tendon and the large muscles you feel on the back of your calf. Good flexibility helps reduce the risk of injury, calf discomfort, and heel pain. The Achilles Stretch is especially helpful for cooling down after walking or cycling and for people with ankylosing spondylitis or psoriatic arthritis. Also do this exercise if you get calf cramps.

1. Stand at a counter or against a wall. Place one foot in front of the other, toes pointing forward and heels on the ground.

2. Lean forward, bend the knee of the forward leg and keep the back knee straight, heel down. You will feel a good stretch in the calf.

3. Hold the stretch for fifteen seconds. *Do not bounce.* Move gently.

It's easy to get sore doing this exercise. If you have worn shoes with high heels for a long time, be particularly careful.

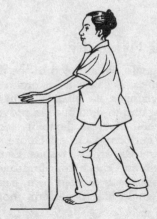

The Whole Body

30. The Stretcher

This exercise is a whole-body stretch to do lying on your back. Start the motion at your ankles as explained here, or reverse the process if you want to start with your arms first.

1. Point your toes, and then pull your toes toward your nose. Relax.

2. Bend your knees. Then flatten your knees and let them relax.

3. Arch your back. Do the Pelvic Tilt (Exercise 16). Relax.

4. Breathe in and stretch your arms above your head. You can raise your arms either to the side or in front of you, whichever feels natural and comfortable. Breathe out and lower your arms. Relax.

5. Stretch your right arm above your head, and stretch your left leg by pushing away from you with your heel. Hold for a count of ten. Switch to the other side and repeat.

Self-Tests for Flexibility

Whatever our goals, we all need to see that our efforts make a difference. Because an exercise program produces gradual changes, it's often hard to tell if the program is working and to recognize improvement.

Choose several of these flexibility tests to measure your progress. Perform each test before you start your exercise program. Record the results. Every four weeks, do the tests again and check your improvement.

Make up some tests of your own, using motions or tasks that you would like to perform more easily, such as reaching a high shelf, tying a shoe, or scratching your back.

Test 1. Arm Flexibility

Do Exercise 6, Pat and Reach (p. 125), for both sides of the body. Ask someone to measure the distance between your fingertips.

Goal: Less distance between your fingertips.

Test 2. Shoulder Flexibility

Stand facing a wall with your toes touching the wall. One arm at a time, reach up the wall in front of you. Hold a pencil and mark the spot or have someone mark how far you reached. Also do this standing sideways, to the wall, about three inches (8 cm) away from the wall.

Goal: To reach higher.

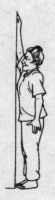 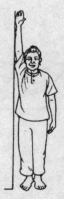

Test 3. Hamstring Flexibility

Do Exercise 24, Hamstring Stretch (page 140), one leg at a time. Keep your thigh perpendicular to your body. How much does your knee bend? How tight does the back of your leg feel?

Goal: Straighter knee and less tension in the back of the leg.

Test 4. Ankle Flexibility

Sit in a chair with your bare feet flat on the floor and your knees bent at a 90-degree angle. Keep your heels on the floor. Raise your toes and the front of your foot. Ask someone to measure the distance between the ball of your foot and the floor.

Goal: One to two inches (3 to 5 cm) between your foot and the floor.

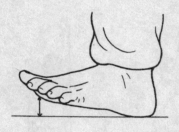

Chapter 11

Strengthening Exercises

The exercises in this chapter make your muscles work against resistance and thus grow stronger. If you are not exercising regularly now, do not start with this chapter. Go to Chapter 10 and begin a program of flexibility exercises. Once you can do flexibility exercises for fifteen consecutive minutes, add strengthening exercises as well as aerobic activity (see Chapter 12). Choose exercises to build a program for the whole body. Always start your exercise session with some flexibility exercises or a short walk to warm up; don't jump straight to strengthening or aerobic activity.

Tips for Strengthening Exercises

This chapter describes exercises for all parts of the body. The exercises for your trunk and legs use gravity, your body weight, or other muscles for resistance. The upper-body exercises use both handheld weights and elastic bands as resistance; choose one of these methods, weights or bands. The exercises that are especially important for posture are labeled "VIP" (very important for posture).

Follow these tips as you plan your program of strengthening exercises:

▼ Start off doing no more than five repetitions.

▼ Gradually increase to no more than ten repetitions of eight to ten different exercises.

▼ Go slowly. Muscle soreness and stiffness often do not show up for twenty-four to forty-eight hours after the exercise.

▼ Always do the same exercises for your left side as for your right.

▼ Breathe naturally. Do not hold your breath. Count out loud to make yourself breathe.

▼ Do strengthening exercises two or three times a week only. Your muscles adapt and get stronger after the exercise, during the rest period, and before you do resistance exercise again. So it is important to give them time to improve.

▼ Eat well-balanced meals to give your muscles the nutrition needed to adapt and strengthen.

Back- and Abdomen-Strengthening Exercises

31. Back Up (VIP)

This exercise strengthens back muscles.

1. Lie on your stomach with your arms at your side or overhead.

2. Lift your head, shoulders, and arms. *Do not look up*. Keep looking down, with your chin tucked in.

3. Count out loud as you hold for a count of ten. Relax.

You can also lift your legs off the floor instead of your head and shoulders.

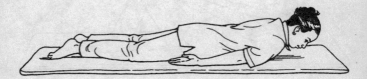

32. Curl-up (VIP)

A Curl-up, as shown here, will strengthen abdominal muscles. Lie on your back, knees bent, feet flat. Do the Pelvic Tilt (Exercise 16). Slowly curl up to raise your head and shoulders. Uncurl back down, or hold for ten seconds and slowly lower your shoulders and head. Keep your chin in.

Breathe out as you curl up, and breathe in as you go back down. *Do not hold your breath.* If you have neck problems or if your neck hurts when you do this exercise, try the next one instead. Never tuck your feet under a chair or have someone hold your feet!

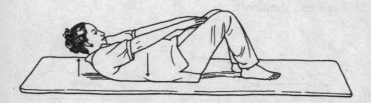

33. Roll-out

This is another good abdominal strengthener and easy on the neck. Use it instead of the Curl-up, or, if neck pain is not a problem, do them both. You strengthen your abdominal muscles by holding a Pelvic Tilt against the weight of your leg. Do not do this exercise if it causes hip or back pain.

1. Lie on your back with knees bent and feet flat. Bring one knee up to your chest.

2. Do the Pelvic Tilt (Exercise 16) and hold your lower back firmly against the floor.

3. Slowly and carefully, move the elevated leg away from your chest as you straighten your knee. Move your leg out until you feel your lower back start to arch.

4. Tuck your knee back to your chest. Reset your pelvic tilt and move your leg out again. Breathe out as your leg moves out. *Do not hold your breath.*

5. Repeat with the other leg.

As you get stronger, you'll be able to straighten your legs out farther.

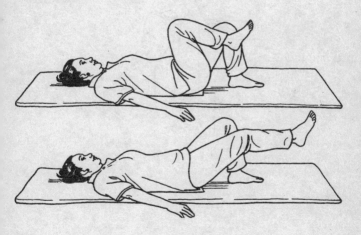

Hip-Strengthening Exercises

34. Back Kick (VIP)

This exercise increases the backward mobility and strength of your hip. Hold on to a counter for support. Move the leg up and back. Keep your knee fairly straight and do not point your toes. Stand tall and do not arch your back.

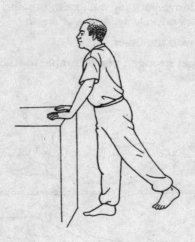

35. Leg Up

This is a good exercise to keep hips strong and in good position.

1. Lying on your stomach, raise one leg at a time up in the air. Use your buttock muscles. Bend the knee slightly if you wish, and keep the foot and ankle relaxed. Pointing your toes and bending your knee at the same time can lead to cramps.

2. Do not roll from side to side. Lower your leg slowly.

3. Raise the other leg. Your back may be more comfortable with a pillow under your stomach. If you are unable to lie on your stomach, you can do the movement standing (Back Kick, Exercise 34).

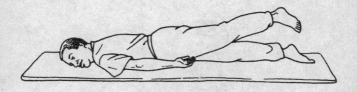

36. Ups and Downs

This is a good exercise to strengthen many muscles in your legs that are important for rising from a chair, climbing stairs, and walking.

1. Standing in front of a chair with arms at your sides or slightly in front of you, slowly bend hips and knees as if you were going to sit down.

2. Lower yourself only halfway, then straighten your hips and knees to stand back up again. Do not use your hands to help.

   Do not lower yourself so far that you can't straighten back up by yourself or so far that your knees hurt. As you get stronger, you will be able to go farther down.

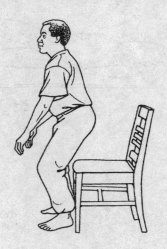

37. Side Kick

This exercise can be done either lying on your side (A) or standing (B). Do it lying down if standing on one leg makes your hip hurt.

A. Lying on your side, bend bottom leg and arm for support. Keep the upper leg straight and in line with your body. Raise the leg up in the air, keeping your knee and toes pointing straight forward. Hold briefly and relax. When you have finished one side, roll over to exercise the other side.

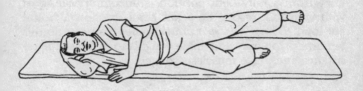

B. Stand using a chair or counter for support. Standing up straight and keeping your leg in line with your body, raise your leg out to the side, keeping knee and toes facing forward. Hold briefly and relax. Repeat on the other side.

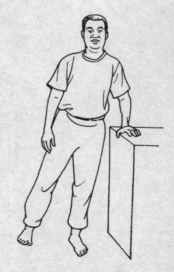

Knee- and Ankle-Strengthening Exercises

38. Knee Strengthener (VIP)

Strong knees are important for walking, stair climbing, getting up and down, and standing comfortably. This exercise strengthens the knee. Sitting in a chair, straighten the knee by tightening up the muscle on top of your thigh. Place your hand on your thigh and feel the muscle work. Hold your knee as straight as possible. As your knee strengthens, see if you can build up to holding your leg out for thirty seconds. If straightening your knee from a fully bent position is uncomfortable, start with your foot resting on a low stool, as shown. Count out loud. *Do not hold your breath.* When you can do this ten times, you may add ankle weights to increase the resistance and make muscles stronger.

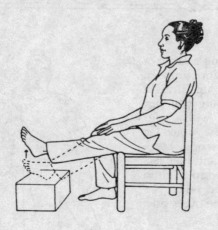

39. Power Knees

This exercise strengthens the muscles that bend and straighten your knee.

1. Sit in a straight-backed chair and cross your legs above the ankles. Your legs can be almost straight, or you can bend your knees as much as you like. Try several positions.

2. Push forward with your back leg and press backward with your front leg. Exert pressure evenly so that your legs do not move.

3. Hold and count out loud for ten seconds. Relax.

4. Change leg positions. Be sure to keep breathing.

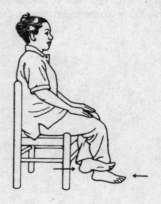

40. Ready-Set-Go

If you have painful knees, this is a good exercise to do when you first stand up.

1. Stand with one foot slightly in front of the other, heel of the forward leg on the ground, and toes off the ground (as if you are going to take a step).

2. Straighten and tighten the knee of the forward leg by tensing the muscles on the front of the thigh. Hold for a count of five. Relax.

3. Say "Go" to yourself each time you tighten the muscles.

Try two or three "Go's" on each knee before you start to walk and then say "Go" to yourself each time your heel touches the floor to remind you to use your knee muscles correctly.

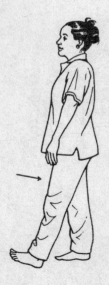

41. Tiptoes

This exercise will help strengthen your calf muscles and make walking, climbing stairs, and standing less tiring.

1. Hold on to a counter or table for support and rise up on your tiptoes. Hold for five seconds.

2. Lower slowly.

How high you go is not as important as keeping your balance and controlling your ankles. It is easier to do both legs at the same time. If your feet are too sore, wear shoes or do it while sitting down.

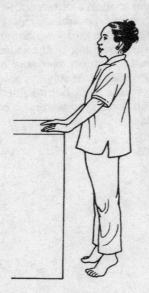

Upper-Body Strengthening Exercises

Upper-Body Strengthening Exercises with Weights

Start with no weights or no more than 0.5 to 3 pounds (0.25 to 1.5 kg). It is better to learn to do the movement correctly before adding weights. You should be able to complete at least eight repetitions with only mild fatigue before adding or increasing weight. Exercise at a comfortable speed. Make sure that you relax after each motion. Count to make the periods of work and relaxation of equal length. Do strengthening exercises within your comfortable range of motion and remember to maintain good posture and normal breathing. Hand weights can be padded to increase the grip size. Some people like wrist weights because grasping is eliminated; however, these can be difficult to slip on over sore hands. Sometimes a homemade weight can solve problems best, for example, socks or plastic soda bottles filled with different amounts of sand, beans, or water, or canned goods of different weights.

42. Upright Row

1. Start with your arms relaxed in front of your body, with your hands together, and the palms facing the body.

2. Lift the hands straight up to chest level. The elbows bend and move out to the side and the hands stay together.

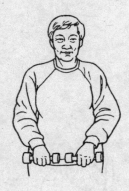 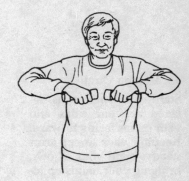

43. Lateral Lift

1. Start with your arms relaxed at your sides, with the palms facing in.

2. Lift your arms up and out to the sides with elbows straight and palms facing down.

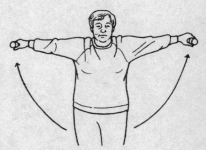

44. Triceps Press

Start with your elbow bent and your hand at your side at waist level. Bend slightly forward at the waist. Keep your upper arm steady and straighten your elbow.

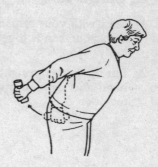

45. Biceps Curl

Start with your arms relaxed at your sides and your palms facing forward. Keeping your upper arms steady, bend your elbows, bringing your hands up toward your shoulders.

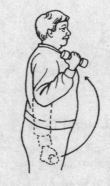

Upper-Body Strengthening with Elastic Bands

Another way to strengthen muscles is to use large elastic bands for resistance. These are available from exercise classes, sports stores, and catalogues. The strength of the resistance varies, and you will want to try out the resistance that is best for you. Move through your comfortable range of motion and make sure you are in control. Do not let the band pull you around. Good posture and natural breathing are important when you do these exercises. A good goal is to gradually build up to repeating each exercise eight to ten times. Bands can be used as loops or with handles. Elastic bands can put a lot of stress on hands and wrists and may not be a good choice for everyone.

46. Horizontal Pull

1. Start with your arms out in front of you at shoulder level, with your elbows and wrists straight. Turn your palms down or facing each other, whichever is more comfortable.

2. Keep your arms at shoulder level and move your hands apart, pulling your arms out to your sides. Relax.

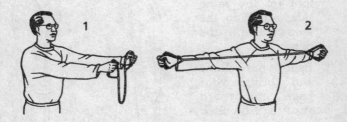

47. Chest Press

1. Place the band across your back, resting it snugly over your shoulder blades. With your elbows bent, hold the ends of the band in front of each underarm. Your thumbs should be up, as when you hold a mug.

2. Straighten your elbows, pressing your arms forward. Relax.

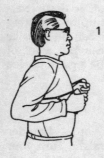
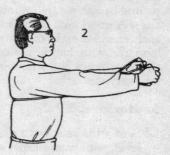

48. Biceps Curl

1. Hold both ends of the band in one hand. Using the foot on the same side, stand on the loop created by the band.

2. Bend your elbow and bring your hand up toward your shoulder. Relax.

3. Repeat with the opposite arm and foot.

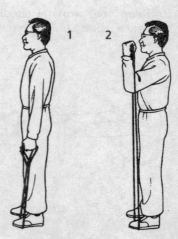

Self-Tests for Strength

We all need to see that our efforts make a difference. Because an exercise program produces gradual change, it's often hard to tell whether the program is working and to recognize improvement. Choose several of these strength tests to measure your progress. Not everyone will be able to do all the tests. Choose those that work best for you. Perform each test before you start your exercise program. Record the results. Every four weeks, do the tests again and check your improvement.

Test 1. Grip Strength

Roll up a blood-pressure cuff and secure it with an elastic bandage or surgical tape. Have someone inflate the cuff to about 30 mm Hg and then squeeze it as hard as you can in your fist. Record the readings for both hands.

Goal: Stronger grip, higher readings.

Test 2. Abdominal Strength

Use Exercise 32, Curl-up (page 150). Count how many repetitions you can do before you get too tired to do more or count how many you can do in thirty seconds.

Goal: More repetitions.

Test 3. Knee and Hip Strength

Count how many times in thirty seconds you can stand up from a chair and sit without using your hands.

Goal: More repetitions, less fatigue.

Ask someone to time you and see how long it takes you to go up and down a flight of steps or walk fifty feet (15 meters).

Goal: Less time, faster speed.

Test 4. Ankle Strength

This test has two parts. Stand at a table or counter for support.

Do Exercise 41, Tiptoes (page 159), as quickly and as often as you can. How many can you do in fifteen seconds?

Stand with your feet flat. Put most of your weight on one foot and quickly tap the front part of your other foot. How many taps can you do in fifteen seconds?

Goal: More repetitions in each movement.

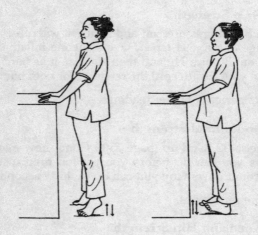

Chapter 12

Aerobic Activities

Who Needs Aerobics?

We all need some aerobic exercise on a regular basis. If you walk, swim, do aquaerobics, bicycle, or walk when you golf, you are doing aerobic exercise. Aerobic exercise is any physical activity that requires you to continuously move your arms or legs for at least five minutes. Regular aerobic exercise helps protect us from heart disease, high blood pressure, and diabetes. Aerobic exercise also helps us to control our weight, sleep well, and feel relaxed, energetic, and happy. This chapter contains suggestions for different kinds of aerobic exercise and ideas for putting together an aerobic exercise program of your own.

If you are not physically active now and have little experience with a regular exercise program, you may want to use the Physical Activity Recommendation for Health data (see page 106) to begin becoming more active. It is not always necessary to add a new or unknown exercise if you can figure out ways to add more physical activity to your current routines. Try adding a five- to ten-minute walk three times a day, maybe with your dog, to get mail or the paper, or to go to the corner store. Once you are able to meet the guidelines for thirty minutes of moderate physical activity on most days of the week, you will probably be looking forward to getting involved in a more formal exercise program.

Your Aerobic Exercise Plan

One of the biggest problems with aerobic exercise is that you may overdo it. Inexperienced exercisers think they have to work very hard for exercise to do any good. Exhaustion, sore muscles, and painful joints are the result of jumping in too hard and too fast. Finding the aerobic exercise plan that is right for you doesn't need to be a guessing game. Use the following guidelines as you plan your aerobic exercise.

The Warm-up

Always warm up before your aerobic exercise. A warm-up raises the temperature in your muscles and joints, increases flexibility, increases circulation, and safely prepares your heart to work harder. A warm-up routine consists of flexibility exercises and a gradual increase in your aerobic activity level. Flexibility exercises prepare your muscles and joints for more vigorous activity and ready your heart and lungs for more work.

A good warm-up routine can consist of ten or fifteen minutes of flexibility exercises and five minutes of easy all-body movements. Examples of the all-body warm-ups are slow walking before a more vigorous aerobic walk, slow dancing before moving to faster music, or pedaling the bicycle at a slower speed and with no resistance before you go on to a more energetic ride.

The Cool-down

A short five- to ten-minute cool-down period after you have finished a more vigorous activity is important to help your body gradually return to a resting state. The cool-down gives your heart a chance to slow down gradually, your body a chance to lose some of the heat you generated during exercise, and your muscles a chance to relax and stretch out.

To cool down, continue your aerobic exercise in slow motion for three to five minutes. For example, after a brisk walk, cool down with a casual stroll. End a bicycle ride with slow, easy pedaling. The cool-down is a good time to do some flexibility exercises because your muscles and joints are warm and less stiff. Gentle flexibility exercises during cool-down help reduce muscle soreness that sometimes follows vigorous activity. If you have been walking or bicycling, be sure to include the Achilles Stretch (Exercise 29, page 143).

Frequency: How Often?
Three or four times a week is the best frequency for aerobic exercise. Taking every other day off gives your body a chance to rest and adapt.

Duration: How Long?
If you have not been active in a while, start your aerobic exercise with no more than five minutes at a time. You can exercise five minutes several times a day and gradually increase the duration of your aerobic activity to about thirty minutes a session or continue to spread exercising out over the day. You can also safely increase the duration of your aerobic exercise by alternating periods of brisk and easy exercise. For example, walk slowly for three to five minutes, then walk briskly for the same amount of time, and then slow down again. Eventually you can build up to longer periods of brisk exercise and use the slow periods as warm-ups and cool-downs.

Intensity: How Hard?
Safe and effective aerobic exercise should be done at no more than moderate intensity. High-intensity exercise increases the risk of injury and causes discomfort, so not many people stick with it. Exercise intensity is measured

by how hard you work. For a trained runner, completing a mile in ten minutes is probably low-intensity exercise. For a person who hasn't exercised in a long time, a brisk ten-minute walk may be moderate to high intensity. The trick, of course, is to figure out what is moderate intensity for you. There are several easy ways to do this.

Perceived Exertion

An easy and reliable way to monitor intensity is to rate how hard you feel you're working on a scale of 0 to 10. Zero, at the low end of the scale, is lying down, doing no work at all. Ten is equivalent to working as hard as possible—very hard work that you couldn't do longer than a few seconds. Of course, you never want to exercise at level 10. A good level for aerobic exercise is between 3 and 5 on this scale. If you are just starting to exercise, stay at 3 or 4.

Heart Rate

Unless you're taking heart-regulating medication, monitoring your pulse while exercising is a good way to measure exercise intensity. The faster the heart beats, the harder you're working. (Your heart also beats fast when you are frightened or nervous, but here we're talking about how your heart responds to physical activity.) Aerobic exercise at moderate intensity raises your heart rate into a range between 60 and 80% of your maximum heart rate. Maximum heart rate declines with age, so your safe exercise heart rate gets lower as you get older. You can use the Suggested Exercise Heart Rate table on page 172 to find your exercise heart rate.

If you want to use heart rate to guide your exercise, you need to know how to take your pulse. You'll need a digital clock or a clock with a second hand. Take your pulse by placing the pads of your middle three fingers at your wrist below the base of your thumb. Don't use the tips of your fingers, and don't use your thumb. You

Perceived Exertion Scale
How Does the Exercise Feel?

Number	Rating
0	Nothing at all
1	Very Weak
2	Weak
3	Moderate
4	Somewhat Strong
5	Strong
6	
7	Very Strong
8	
9	
10	Very, Very Strong

should be able to feel your blood pumping. Count how many beats you feel in fifteen seconds. Multiply this number by 4 to find out how fast your heart is beating in one minute. Start taking your pulse whenever you think of it, and you'll soon learn the difference between your resting and exercise heart rates.

The most important reason for knowing your exercise heart rate range is so that you can learn not to exercise too vigorously. After you've done your warm-up and five minutes of aerobic activity, take your pulse. If it's higher than the upper rate on the chart, slow down. Don't work so hard. If you are a beginning exerciser, keep your exercise heart rate down at the lower end of the range shown on the Suggested Exercise Heart Rate table.

Suggested Exercise Heart Rate, by Age

Age Range	Pulse (Number of Heartbeats in 15 Seconds)
20–30	30–38
30–40	28–36
40–50	26–34
50–60	24–32
60–70	22–30
70–80	20–28
80+	18–24

At first some people have trouble getting their heart rate up to the lower rate. Don't worry about that. Keep exercising at a comfortable level. As you get more experienced and stronger, your heart rate will rise, because you can exercise more vigorously.

If you are taking medicine that regulates your heart rate, have trouble feeling your pulse, or think that keeping track of your heart rate is a bother, use one of the other methods to monitor your exercise intensity.

Talk Test

Talk to another person or yourself or recite poems while you exercise. Moderate-intensity exercise allows you to speak comfortably. If you can't carry on a conversation because you are breathing too hard or are short of breath, you're working too hard. Slow down. The talk test is an easy way to regulate exercise intensity.

Remember to follow the guidelines on frequency, duration, and intensity of exercise. Sometimes you need to tell yourself (and maybe others) that enough is enough.

More exercise is not necessarily better, especially if it gives you pain or discomfort. As the *Walking Magazine* said, "Go for the smiles, not the miles."

Walking

You can walk to condition your heart and lungs, strengthen bones and muscles, relieve tension, control weight, and generally feel good. Walking is easy, inexpensive, safe, and accessible. You can walk by yourself or with company, and you can take your exercise with you wherever you go. Walking is safer and less stressful than jogging or running. It's an especially good choice if you have been sedentary or have joint problems.

Most people with arthritis, even knee arthritis, can walk as a fitness activity. If you walk to shop, visit friends, and do household chores, then you'll probably be able to walk for exercise. Using a cane or walker need not stop you from getting into a walking routine. If you are in a wheelchair, use crutches, or experience more than mild discomfort when you walk a short distance, you should consider some other type of aerobic exercise, or consult a physician or therapist for help.

Be cautious during the first two weeks of walking. If you haven't been doing much for a while, ten minutes of walking may be enough. Build up your time with intervals of strolling. Each week increase the brisk walking interval by no more than five minutes until you are up to twenty or thirty minutes. Follow the frequency, duration, and intensity guidelines, and read the tips below on walking before you start.

Walking Tips
1. **Choose your ground.** Walk on a flat, level surface. Walking on hills, uneven ground, soft earth, sand, or gravel is hard work and often leads to hip, knee, or foot pain. Fitness trails, shopping malls, school

tracks, streets with sidewalks, and quiet neighborhoods are good places to get started.

2. **Always warm up and cool down with a stroll.** It's important to walk slowly for three to five minutes to prepare your circulation and muscles for a brisk walk and to finish up with the same slow walk to let your body slow down gradually. Experienced walkers know they can avoid shin and foot discomfort when they begin and end with a stroll.

3. **Set your own pace.** It takes practice to find the right walking speed. To find your speed, start walking slowly for a few minutes, then increase your speed to a pace that is slightly faster than normal for you. After five minutes, take your pulse and see if you are within your exercise heart rate range. If you are above the range or feel out of breath, slow down. If you are below the range, try walking a little faster. Walk another five minutes and take your pulse again. If you are still below your exercise range, don't try to raise your heart rate by walking uncomfortably fast. Keep walking at a comfortable speed and take your pulse in the middle and at the end of each walk.

4. **Increase your arm work.** You can also raise your heart rate into exercise range by bending your elbows a bit and swinging your arms more vigorously. Alternatively, carry a one- or two-pound (0.5 to 1 kg) weight in each hand. You can purchase hand weights for walking; hold a can of food in each hand; or put sand, dried beans, or pennies in two small plastic beverage bottles or socks. The extra work you do with your arms increases your heart rate without forcing you to walk faster than you find comfortable.

5. **Use knee flexibility and strengthening exercises if you have knee pain.** If your knees hurt or you have increased discomfort after you start walking, try

knee flexibility exercises before and after you walk and add some strengthening exercises three days a week.

Shoes

It's not necessary to spend a lot of money on shoes. Wear shoes of the correct length and width with shock-absorbing soles and insoles. Make sure they're big enough in the toe area: The "rule of thumb" is a thumb width between the end of your longest toe and the end of the shoe. You shouldn't feel pressure on the sides or tops of your toes. The shoe should hold your heel firmly when you walk so your heel doesn't slip up and down.

Wear shoes with a continuous crepe or composite sole in good repair. Shoes with leather soles and a separate heel don't absorb shock as well as the newer athletic and casual shoes. Shoes with laces or Velcro let you adjust width as needed and give more support than slip-ons. If you have problems tying laces, consider Velcro closures or elastic shoelaces.

Many people like shoes with removable insoles that can be exchanged for ones that are more shock absorbing. Insoles are available in sporting goods stores and shoe stores. When you shop for insoles, take your walking shoes with you. Try on the shoe with the insole to make sure that there's still enough room inside for your foot to be comfortable. Insoles come in sizes and can be trimmed with scissors for a final fit. If your toes take up extra room, try the three-quarter insoles that stop just short of your toes. If you have prescribed inserts in your shoes already, ask your doctor, therapist, or orthotist about insoles.

Possible Problems

1. If you have pain around your shins when you walk, you may not be spending enough time warming up.

Do the ankle flexibility and strengthening exercises (pages 141–143 and 156–159) before you start walking. Start your walk at a slow pace for at least five minutes. Keep your feet and toes relaxed.

2. Another common problem is sore knees. Fast walking puts more stress on knee joints. To slow your speed and keep your heart rate up, try doing more work with your arms (see number 4 under "Walking Tips" above). Do the knee-strengthening exercises (exercises 38 and 39, pages 156–157) in your warm-up to help reduce knee pain.

3. Cramps in the calf and heel pain can often be eliminated by doing the Achilles Stretch (Exercise 29, page 143) before and after walking. A slow walk to warm up also is helpful. If you have circulatory problems in your legs and experience cramps while walking, alternate intervals of brisk and slow walking. If this doesn't help, check with your physician or therapist for suggestions. Dehydration can also cause leg cramps. Make sure you increase your fluid intake while exercising.

4. Maintain good posture. Use the chin-in position (Exercise 1, page 121) and keep your shoulders relaxed to help reduce neck and upper-back discomfort.

Swimming

Swimming is another good aerobic exercise. The buoyancy of the water lets you move your joints through their full range of motion and strengthen your muscles and cardiovascular system with less joint stress than on land. Swimming uses the whole body. If you haven't been swimming for a while, consider a refresher course.

To make swimming an aerobic exercise, you will eventually need to swim continuously for twenty minutes. Use the frequency, duration, and intensity guidelines to build up your endurance. Try different strokes, modifying them or changing strokes after each lap or two. This lets you exercise all joints and muscles without overtiring any one area.

Swimming Tips

1. **Use a mask and snorkel for breathing.** The breast stroke and crawl require a lot of neck motion and may be uncomfortable if you have neck pain. To solve this problem, use a mask and snorkel to breathe without twisting your neck.

2. **Use swim goggles to protect eyes.** Chlorine can be irritating to eyes. A good pair of goggles will protect your eyes and let you keep your eyes open while you're swimming.

3. **Take a hot shower or soak in a hot tub after your workout.** The warmth helps reduce stiffness and muscle soreness that may come from being in cool water.

4. **Always swim where there are qualified lifeguards.**

If you don't like to swim or are uncomfortable learning strokes, you can walk laps in the pool or join the millions who are aquacizing.

Aquacize

Exercising in the water is comfortable, fun, and effective as a flexibility, strengthening, and aerobic activity. The buoyancy of the water takes weight off hips, knees, feet, and back. People who have trouble walking for endurance can usually aquacize. The pool is a good place to do your own routine, because no one can see you much below shoulder level.

Getting Started

Joining a water exercise class with a good instructor is an excellent way to get started. The Arthritis Foundation and Arthritis Society sponsor water exercise classes and train instructors. Contact your local chapter or branch office to see what is available. Many communities and private health clubs offer water exercise classes, with some geared to older adults.

If you have access to a pool and want to exercise on your own, there are many water exercise books available. One we recommend is *HydroRobics* (by Joseph A. Krasevec and Diane C. Grimes, Human Kinetics, 1985), which contains good ideas for exercise in the water.

Water temperature is always a topic when people talk about water exercise. The U.S. Arthritis Foundation recommends a pool temperature of 84°F (29°C) with the surrounding air temperature in the same range. Except in warm climates, this means a heated pool. If you're just starting to aquacize, find a pool with these temperatures. If you can exercise more vigorously and don't have Raynaud's phenomenon or other cold sensitivity, you can probably aquacize in cooler water. Many pools where people swim laps are about 80°F to 83°F (27°C to 28°C). It feels quite cool when you first get in, but starting off with water walking, jogging, or another whole-body exercise helps you warm up quickly.

The deeper the water you stand in, the less stress there is on joints; however, a water level above midchest can make it hard to keep your balance. You can let the water cover more of your body just by spreading your legs apart or bending your knees a bit.

Aquacize Tips

1. **Protect your feet.** Wear something on your feet to protect them from rough pool floors and to provide traction in the pool and on the deck. Choices vary from terry cloth slippers with rubber soles (they

stretch in water, so buy a size smaller than your shoe size) to footgear especially designed for water exercise. Some styles have Velcro to make them easier to put on. Beach shoes with rubber soles and mesh tops also work well. Do not wear thong sandals around or in a pool.

2. **Keep warm.** If you are sensitive to cold or have Raynaud's phenomenon, wear a pair of disposable latex surgical gloves. Boxes of gloves are available at most pharmacies. The water trapped and warmed inside the glove seems to insulate the hand. If your body gets cold in the water, wear a T-shirt, full-leg Lycra exercise tights, or both for warmth.

3. **Try a step stool for easier access.** If the pool does not have steps and it is difficult for you to climb up and down a ladder, try positioning a three-step kitchen stool in the pool by the ladder rails. This is an inexpensive way to provide steps for easier entry and exit, and it is easy to remove and store when not needed.

4. **Add more buoyancy.** Wearing a flotation belt or life vest adds extra buoyancy, to take weight off hips, knees, and feet, and makes exercising more comfortable for these joints.

5. **Regulate exercise intensity.** You can regulate how hard you work in the water by how you move. To make the work easier, move more slowly. Another way to regulate exercise intensity is to change how much water you push when you move. For example, when you move your arms back and forth in front of you under water, it is hard work if you hold your palms facing each other and clap. It is easier if you turn your palms down and slice your arms back and forth with only the narrow edge of your hands pushing against the water.

Bicycling

Outdoor Bicycling

Cyclists who travel outdoors can enjoy the scenery and get out into the fresh air and sunshine. But they also face the risks of streets and bike paths, especially the danger of falling. Falls from bicycles can be serious. If you have problems with balance, vision, or hearing, or if you have osteoporosis, outdoor bicycling may not be for you. Consider a stationary bicycle instead (see the next section).

If you live in a flat area, consider an adult tricycle. Though heavy and harder to pedal than a bicycle, tricycles are very stable. These tricycles typically feature a large basket that makes it easy to carry packages and run errands.

Finding the Right Bicycle

A bicycle that is the proper size for you, and that is properly adjusted, is essential. Incorrect seat height is the most common problem. It is also the easiest adjustment to make. To check seat height, have someone hold the bike while you sit on the seat. With your *heel* on the pedal, straighten your leg to the bottom of the pedal stroke. If your knee is still bent, the seat is too low. Keeping your knees bent while pedaling can cause knee pain. (People whose knees bend backward should leave just a little bend.) If you can't keep your heel on the pedal when the pedal is at its lowest point, you need to lower the seat.

Try different kinds of handlebars, gears, and brakes to find the styles that suit you best. Many bicycle shops can customize a bike by combining the features you want. Reading, talking to other bicyclists, and taking a trip to a bike shop will help you decide on your kind of bike. Once you know the features you want, you may be able to find what you want at a yard sale or through a classified ad. Just get a professional safety check and tune-up before you ride.

Whatever style you choose, remember that bicycling uses different muscles from walking. Don't be surprised if a five- or ten-minute ride is enough at first. Follow the guidelines of frequency, duration, and intensity to progress gradually to twenty or thirty minutes of safe and enjoyable bicycling.

Riding Tips

1. **Wear a helmet.** The most important piece of equipment for bicycle riding is a helmet. Any fall can cause serious head injury. Don't risk it. There are ventilated helmets that weigh less than eight ounces (227 g). Look for a sticker showing that the helmet has been approved by a safety board, such as Snell or ANSI in the United States.

2. **Follow the rules.** Learn and obey the bicycle road rules for your community. Take advantage of roads with a designated bicycle lane.

3. **Pedal with the *ball* of your foot.**

4. **Use gears correctly for safety and comfort.** Learn to use your gears so that you don't grind them. If you work hard to pedal and start to feel pain around your kneecap, you probably need to shift to a lower gear.

Stationary Bicycles

Stationary bicycles offer the fitness benefits of outdoor bicycling without the outdoor hazards. They're preferable for people who don't have the flexibility or strength to be comfortable pedaling and steering on the road. If you live in a cold or hilly area, you may want to avoid the extra exertion of cycling outdoors. Stationary bicycling is good when combined with other kinds of aerobic exercise to provide choices between indoor and outdoor, solitary and group, and weight-bearing and nonweight-bearing exercise.

Choosing a Bicycle

A wide variety of stationary bicycles is available. Most models have a speedometer and odometer to show the speed and distance. Some take your pulse by means of a chest strap or hand grips and give a digital readout. Models at health clubs may have computer programs and video displays to take you over hills and dales. There are also recumbent bicycles that place hips and knees at about the same height. Some people find these the most comfortable.

Important features that differ from model to model include the following:

1. **Seat.** Both regular bicycle and larger, flatter bench-style seats are available. Seats can be adjusted vertically or both vertically and horizontally. Adjust the seat so that your knee is straight when your *heel* is on the pedal at the pedal's lowest point. If your knees are unstable or loose or bend backward, adjust the seat height so that there is a little bend left in your knee, rather than having your legs be completely straight. If your knees don't straighten all the way, adjust the seat so that they are comfortably straight.

2. **Handlebars.** Stationary handlebars are for balance and for supporting your arms. Movable handlebars let you exercise the upper body. Using your arms as you exercise helps you spread the work out instead of depending on your legs to do it all. You should be able to grip the handlebars without reaching or stretching and with a slight bend in your elbows.

3. **Resistance.** How hard you have to push to turn the pedals can be adjusted with a dial or screw. On some models a fan wheel increases resistance as you pedal

faster. If the resistance adjustment is manual, make sure you can easily reach and turn the control.

A loan or rental is a good way to start using a stationary bicycle. The classified ads are a great place to shop for your own. Not all models fit everyone, so try out any bicycle you are considering. Make sure it adjusts to positions that are comfortable and safe for you. Check all the points listed below.

▼ The bicycle is steady when you get on and off.

▼ The resistance is easy to set and can be set to zero.

▼ The seat is comfortable.

▼ The seat can be adjusted for full knee extension when the pedal is at its lowest point.

▼ The pedals are large enough and the pedal straps loose enough to allow feet to shift easily while you are pedaling.

▼ There is ample clearance from the frame for knees and ankles.

▼ The handlebars allow good posture and comfortable arm position.

Make It Interesting

The most common complaint about riding a stationary bike is that it's boring. If you ride while watching television, reading, or listening to music, you can become fit without being bored. One woman keeps interested by mapping out tours of places she would like to visit, and then she charts her progress on the map as she rolls off the miles. Other people set their bicycle time for the half hour of soap opera or news that they watch every day. There are videocassettes of exotic bike tours that put you in the rider's perspective. Book racks that clip onto the handlebars make reading easy.

Riding Tips

1. **Don't use too much resistance.** Bicycling uses different muscles from walking. Until your leg muscles get used to pedaling, you may be able to ride only a few minutes. Start off with no resistance. If you wish, increase resistance slightly every two weeks. Increasing resistance has the same effect as bicycling up hills. If you use too much resistance, your knees are likely to hurt, and you'll have to stop before you get the benefit of an aerobic exercise.

2. **Pedal at a comfortable speed.** For most people, fifty to sixty revolutions per minute (rpm) is a good place to start. Some bicycles tell you the rpm, or you can count the number of times your right foot reaches its lowest point in a minute. As you get used to bicycling, you can increase your speed. However, faster is not necessarily better. Listening to music at the right tempo makes it easier to pedal at a consistent speed. Experience will tell you the best combination of speed and resistance.

3. **Progress gradually at moderate intensity.** Set your goal for twenty to thirty minutes of pedaling at a comfortable speed. Build up your time by alternating intervals of brisk pedaling with less exertion. Use your heart rate, perceived exertion, or the talk test to make sure you aren't working too hard. If you're alone, try singing songs as you pedal. If you get out of breath, slow down.

4. **Chart progress.** Keep a record of the times and distances of your "bike trips." You'll be amazed at how much you can do.

5. **Keep the exercise habit.** On bad days, or if you have a painful knee, keep your exercise habit going by pedaling with no resistance, at fewer rpm, or for a shorter period.

The stationary bicycle is a particularly good alternative exercise. It does not put weight on your hips, knees, and feet; you can easily adjust how hard you work; and weather doesn't matter. Use the bicycle on days when you don't want to walk, do more vigorous exercise, or can't exercise outside.

Other Exercise Equipment

If you have trouble getting on or off a stationary bicycle or don't have room for a bicycle where you live, you might try a restorator or arm crank. To purchase one, ask your therapist or doctor, or call a medical equipment supplier.

A restorator is a small piece of equipment with foot pedals that can be attached to the foot of a bed or a chair. It allows you to exercise by pedaling. Resistance can be varied, and placement of the restorator lets you adjust for leg length and knee bend. The restorator can be the first step in getting an exercise program started.

Arm cranks are bicycles for the arms. They are mounted on a table. People who are unable to use their legs for active exercise can improve their cardiovascular fitness by using the arm crank. It's important to work closely with a therapist to set up your program because using only your arms for aerobic exercise requires different intensity monitoring from using the bigger leg muscles.

There is a wide variety of exercise equipment in addition to what we've mentioned so far. These include treadmills (self-powered and motor-driven), rowing machines, cross-country skiing machines, minitrampolines, and stair-climbing machines. Most are available in both commercial and home models. If you're thinking about exercise equipment, have your objectives clearly in mind. For cardiovascular fitness and endurance, you want equipment that will help you exercise as much of your body at one time as possible. The motion should be rhythmical, repetitive, and continuous. The equipment should be comfortable, safe, and not stressful on joints. If you're interested in a new piece of equipment, try it out for a week or two before buying it.

Exercise equipment that requires you to use weights usually does not improve cardiovascular fitness. A weight-lifting program builds strength, but it can put excessive stress on joints, muscles, tendons, and ligaments if done incorrectly. It is extremely important that you confer with your doctor or therapist when planning any program that uses weights or weight machines.

Low-Impact Aerobic Dance

Most people find low-impact aerobic dance a safe and acceptable form of exercise. "Low impact" means that one foot is always on the floor and there is no jumping. However, low impact does not necessarily mean low intensity, nor do the low-impact routines protect all joints. If you participate in a low-impact aerobic dance class, you'll probably need to make some modifications for your arthritis. Observe and participate in classes with different instructors to find a class and leader who feel, sound, and look right for you.

Getting Started

Start off by letting the instructor know who you are, that you may modify some movements to meet your needs, and that you may need to ask for advice. It's easier to start off with a newly formed class than to join an ongoing class. If you don't know people, try to get acquainted. Be open about why you may sometimes do things a little differently. You'll be more comfortable and may find others who also have special needs.

Most instructors use music or count to a specific beat and do a set number of repetitions. You may find that the movement is too fast or that you don't want to do as many repetitions. Modify the routine by slowing down to half-time, or keep up with the beat until you start to tire and then slow down. If the class is doing an exercise that involves arms and legs and you get tired, try resting your arms and only doing the leg movements or just walk in place until you are ready to go again. Most instructors will be able to instruct you in "chair aerobics" if you need some time off your feet.

Many low-impact routines use lots of arm movements done at or above shoulder level to raise heart rates. For people who have shoulder problems or high blood pressure, too much arm exercise above shoulder level can cause problems. Modify the exercise by lowering your arms or giving your arms frequent rests.

Being different from the group in a room walled with mirrors takes courage, conviction, and a sense of humor. The most important thing you can do for yourself is to choose an instructor who encourages everyone to exercise at his or her own pace and a class where people are friendly and having fun. Observe classes, speak with instructors, and participate in at least one class session before making any financial commitment.

Aerobic Studio Tips

1. **Wear supportive shoes.** Many studios have cushioned floors and soft carpeting that might tempt you to go barefoot. Don't! Shoes help protect the small joints and muscles in your feet and ankles by providing a firm, flat surface on which to stand.

2. **Protect your knees.** Stand with knees straight but relaxed. Many low-impact routines are done with bent, tensed knees and a lot of bobbing up and down. This can be painful and is unnecessarily stressful to your knees. Avoid this by remembering to keep your knees relaxed (aerobics instructors call this "soft"

knees). Watch in the mirror to see that you keep the top of your head steady as you exercise. Don't bob up and down.

3. **Don't overstretch.** The beginning (warm-up) and end (cool-down) of the session will have stretching and strengthening exercises. Remember to stretch only as far as you comfortably can. Hold the position and don't bounce. If the stretch hurts, don't do it. Ask your instructor for a less stressful substitute or choose one of your own.

4. **Change movements.** Do this often enough so that you don't get sore muscles or joints. It's normal to feel some new sensations in your muscles and around your joints when you start a new exercise program. However, if you feel discomfort doing the same movement for some time, change movements or stop for a while and rest.

5. **Alternate kinds of exercise.** Many exercise facilities have a variety of exercise opportunities: equipment rooms with cardiovascular machines, pools, and aerobic studios. If you have trouble with an hour-long aerobic class, see if you can join the class for the warm-up and cool-down and use a stationary bicycle or treadmill for your aerobic portion. Many people have found that this routine gives them the benefits of both an individualized program and group exercise.

Self-Tests for Aerobic Fitness

It's important to see that your exercise program is making a measurable difference. Choose one of these aerobic fitness tests to perform before you start your exercise program. Pick the test that works best for you. Record your results. After four weeks of exercise, do the test again and check your improvement. Measure yourself after four more weeks. For ideas on other self-tests, see the book *If It Hurts, Don't Do It,* listed under "References" at the end of this chapter.

Test 1. Distance Test

Find a place to walk or bicycle where you can measure distance. A running track works well. On a street you can measure distance with a car. A stationary bicycle with an odometer provides the equivalent measurement. If you plan on swimming, you can count lengths of the pool.

After a warm-up, note your starting point and either bicycle, swim, or walk as briskly as you comfortably can for five minutes. Try to move at a steady pace for the full time. At the end of five minutes, measure and record the distance, your heart rate, and your perceived exertion from 0 to 10. Continue at a slow pace for three to five more minutes to cool down.

Repeat the test after several weeks of exercise. There may be a change in as little as four weeks. However, it often takes eight to twelve weeks to see improvement.

Goal: To cover more distance *or* to lower your heart rate *or* to lower your perceived exertion.

Test 2. Time Test

Measure a given distance you intend to walk, bike, or swim. Estimate how far you think you can go in about five minutes. You can pick a number of blocks, an actual distance measured in feet, or lengths in a pool.

Spend three to five minutes warming up. Then, start timing and start moving steadily, briskly, and comfortably. At the finish, record how long it took you to cover your course, your heart rate, and your perceived exertion.

Repeat after several weeks of exercise. You may see changes in as soon as four weeks. However, it often takes eight to twelve weeks for improvement.

Goal: To complete the course in less time *or* to lower your heart rate *or* to lower your perceived exertion.

Chapter 13

Managing a Healthy Weight

Attaining and maintaining a healthy weight is especially important for people with arthritis. Your weight can have a considerable impact on your disease symptoms, and your ability to exercise or to otherwise manage your disease. Therefore, finding a healthy weight and maintaining it are central elements of the self-management process. But what is a healthy weight?

What it *isn't* is a specific "ideal" weight such as those commonly found in weight tables. Ideal weights in tables are only guidelines based on population statistics. They are not meant to be used to determine a healthy weight. Being at a healthy weight does not mean being thin or skinny like popular images portrayed in the media. Being at a very low weight is unrealistic, if not unachievable, and at the very least is not sustainable for the vast majority of people. Indeed, being too thin can be just as bad for your health as being too fat. Moreover, you should think in terms of a healthy weight range; nearly all of us will vary up and down a few pounds, and that is all right.

Aim for a healthy weight range. This can be a range of about three to five pounds, which you should be able to realistically maintain, where you feel good both mentally and physically, and where you reduce your risk of developing health problems or further complicating existing ones. Determining your healthy weight range depends on several factors, including your body composition (i.e., how much of your body weight is fat), your body fat distribution (i.e., how the fat is distributed on your body), and whether you have weight-related medical problems such as high blood pressure. When you take these things into consideration, you may find that you are already at a healthy weight and need only to maintain it by eating properly and staying active.

If you aren't certain if you are at a healthy weight, an easy way to decide is to figure out your Body Mass Index (BMI). This is a measure of body weight that is based on weight and height and is highly related to health. To figure out your BMI, multiply your weight in pounds by 705 and then divide that by your height in inches squared. For example, if you are 150 lbs and 67 inches tall, then your BMI is 150 lbs. x 705 = 105,750, divided by (67" x 67") = 4489, which equals (105,750/ 4489) = 23.6. According to the following guidelines, your weight is within a healthy weight range.

If your BMI is:

▼ less than 19—this classifies you as being underweight, although this may not be a problem unless there are other health problems.

▼ 19 to 25—this classifies you at a healthy weight.

▼ 26 to 29—this classifies you as being overweight. However, if you are physically active and have a lot of muscle mass, the excess weight may not be due to body fat and so may not be a problem.

▼ 30 to 39—this classifies you as obese, and very likely you have a large amount of body fat.

▼ Over 40—this classifies you as being morbidly obese with a very high proportion of the excess weight being body fat, and it puts you at very high risk of health complications.

Here is a tip for losing weight. Every day add exercise that uses 100 calories (about a half hour) to your usual activities and reduce what you eat by 100 calories (about a cookie or a piece of bread). Over a year this adds up to a 20-pound weight loss.

If you are overweight, consider asking your doctor to refer you to a registered dietitian for help in determining a healthy weight for you, given your condition and treatment needs.

1. Why Change My Weight?

The reasons for losing or gaining weight are different for each individual. The most obvious reason may be your physical health, but there may also be psychological or emotional reasons for wanting to change. Examine why you want to change.

2. What Will I Have to Change?

Two ingredients for successful weight management are developing an active lifestyle and making changes in your eating patterns. Let's look closely at what each of these involves.

An active lifestyle involves physical activity, which burns calories and regulates appetite and metabolism, both important for weight management. Physical activity can also help you develop more strength and stamina, as well as move and breathe more easily. In other words, activity doesn't wear you down or out, but actually boosts your energy level. You will find more information about this and tips for choosing activities that suit your needs and lifestyle in chapters 9, 10, 11, and 12.

While many people are concerned with losing weight and keeping it off, some people with arthritis struggle to gain and maintain a healthy weight. If you experience a continual or extreme weight loss because your disease or medications interfere with your appetite or deplete your body of valuable nutrients (such as proteins, vitamins, and minerals), you may need to work at gaining weight. A registered dietician can advise you on healthful ways to do this.

Making changes in your eating patterns starts by making small, gradual changes in what you eat. For example, begin by reducing the fat and increasing the fiber content in the foods you select. Foods that are high in fiber and low in fat help with weight management, help reduce cholesterol, and prevent constipation and some forms of cancer. The list of "Food Choices" (below) offers some hints for reducing the fat and increasing the fiber in your eating plan. You can find additional information on healthy eating in the references listed at the end of this chapter.

If you decide to increase the amount of fiber you eat, do so gradually. Changing too quickly may overwhelm your digestive system, causing problems with gas, discomfort, or constipation. To prevent constipation, follow the tips on pages 239–242.

Food Choices

Hints for Increasing Fiber

▼ Eat a wide variety of fruits and vegetables.

▼ Eat low-fat, whole-grain products, including breads, hot or cold cereals, crackers, brown rice, and other whole grains.

▼ Drink plenty of water to help move the fiber through.

▼ Try cooked dried beans, peas, and lentils as a substitute for meat—for example, baked beans or split pea or lentil soup.

Hints for Reducing Fat

▼ Eat moderate-size portions of meat, poultry, and fish—2 to 3 oz (50 to 100 g) or about the size of a deck of cards or the palm of your hand.

▼ Choose leaner cuts of meat.

▼ Trim off fat and remove the skin from poultry.

▼ Broil, barbecue, or roast meats instead of frying them.

▼ Skim fat off stews and soups. This is easier if the stew has been refrigerated overnight.

▼ Use low-fat or nonfat (skim) milk and milk products.

▼ Use nonstick pans and a moderate amount of cooking oil spray.

▼ Use added fats like butter, margarine, oils, gravy, sauces, and salad dressings sparingly in food preparation, no more than 3 to 4 teaspoons (15 to 20 ml) per day.

▼ Snack on fruit or nonfat yogurt, instead of cookies or ice cream.

3. Am I Ready to Change?

Success is important in weight management. Therefore, the next step is to evaluate whether you are ready to make these changes. If you are not ready, you may be setting yourself up for failure and frustration because of "yo-yo" dieting. This is when your weight goes up and down. This is not only discouraging but unhealthy. It is helpful to plan ahead by considering the following types of questions:

▼ Is there someone or something that will make it easier for you to change?

▼ Are there problems or obstacles that will keep you from becoming more active or changing the way you eat?

▼ Will worries or concerns about family, friends, work, or other commitments affect your ability to carry out your plans successfully at this time?

Looking at these factors first can help you find ways to build support for making desired changes and to minimize the problems you may encounter along the way.

After you have examined these lists, you may find that now is not the right time to start anything. If it is not, set a date in the future when you will reevaluate. In the meantime, accept that you have made the right decision for you at this time and focus on other goals.

If you decide that now is the right time, start by changing those things that feel most comfortable to you. You don't have to do it all right away. Slow and steady wins the race.

To help get started, keep track of what you are currently doing. For example, write down your daily routine to identify where you might be able to add some exercise. Or keep a food diary for a week to see what and how much you eat, how it's prepared, when and why you are eating. This can help you identify how and where to make changes in your eating patterns, as well as how to shop for and prepare your meals. It may also help you determine if there is any association between your eating patterns and your symptoms. Next, choose only one or two things to change first. For example, if you find you are eating red meat three or four times per week and you tend to fry it, you may want to try broiling it instead. Or you might buy leaner cuts of meat and substitute fish or poultry for some meals. After you have allowed yourself time to get used to these changes, you can then add more. The goal-setting and action-planning skills discussed in Chapter 6 can help you do this.

Part V
Solving Particular Problems

Chapter 14

Pain Management

Pain is a problem shared by most people with arthritis and fibromyalgia. In fact, it is often their number one concern. While pain is a common symptom, each person's experience of pain is unique and quite personal. Pain often is not easy to describe nor can it be seen by others. Therefore, it can be difficult to understand, treat, and manage.

However, by recognizing the multiple factors that contribute to the pain experienced by people with arthritis and fibromyalgia, it is possible to find different techniques to help manage the pain better. Some of these factors include:

▼ *Inflammation and damage in or around the joints and surrounding tissues.*

▼ *Tense and weak muscles.* For people with arthritis, the body's natural response is to protect a painful joint by tensing the muscles around that area. When the muscles are tensed, lactic acid builds up in the muscles, and after a while this buildup also causes pain. In addition, people tend to limit the use of painful joints, which weakens the muscles that support the joint and contributes to the pain. For people with fibromyalgia, a widespread type of muscle tension is actually one of the major features of the condition and a reason for the pain.

▼ *Lack of sleep or a poor quality of sleep.* Pain often interferes with sleep, keeping people from getting either enough sleep or good quality sleep. This, in turn, makes pain and the ability to cope with it worse. This is especially true for people with fibromyalgia.

▼ *Stress, anxiety, and emotions such as depression, anger, fear, and frustration.* These are normal responses to living with a chronic condition like arthritis or fibromyalgia, and they do affect the perception of pain. When someone is stressed, angry, afraid, or depressed, everything, including pain, seems worse.

Because pain can come from many sources, the methods we use to manage or reduce pain must be aimed at all of these different sources. We discuss a variety of such methods not only in this chapter but throughout the book. For instance, exercise that both strengthens and relaxes muscles should be a part of a pain management program (see chapters 9, 10, 11, and 12). Healthy eating is also important in providing the body with energy to combat fatigue and in maintaining a proper weight. One of the best ways to relieve pain in your back, hips, knees, ankles, and feet is to reduce the pressure and stress that extra pounds place on these joints (see Chapter 13). Use of assistive devices, such as a cane or walking stick or long- or large-handled tools can also help relieve pain (see chapters 7 and 8). Understanding and identifying ways to overcome anger, fear, and depression that aggravate pain, as well as ways to express these feelings that affect our relationships with others, are also important parts of a pain management program (see Chapter 16). Lastly, it is important to work with your health-care provider to determine how best to use medications to help you control symptoms (see chapters 17 and 18). These steps, along with the techniques described in this chapter, are all important parts of a self-management program.

This chapter describes a number of simple pain-management techniques that you can practice almost anytime. Some you may have heard of, such as the use of heat or cold to reduce pain in particular joints. We also describe cognitive pain-management techniques. These help you to use the mind in different ways to help relax muscles, reduce stress and anxiety, and decrease pain.

All of us at one time or another have experienced the power of the mind and its effect on the body. For example, when we are embarrassed, we might feel flushed and our face blushes. If we think about sucking on a lemon, our mouth puckers and starts to water. These simple examples illustrate the ability of our thoughts and feelings to affect our bodies. With training and practice, we can learn to use the mind effectively to relieve pain and other symptoms associated with arthritis. In fact, we know from our experiences with many people that these cognitive techniques are powerful self-management tools. In the following pages, we describe several of these techniques.

The following suggestions may help you to use these techniques more effectively.

▼ Try several different techniques to find the ones you like best. Be sure you give each technique a fair trial. This means at least two weeks of practice for a minimum of fifteen to twenty minutes a day before you decide if it is going to be helpful.

▼ Once you have found the techniques you like, think how you will use each one. For example, some exercises can be done anywhere while others require a quiet place. The best pain managers use a variety of techniques that can be mixed and matched to the situations in their daily lives.

▼ To help you get in the habit of using these techniques consistently, try including them in your weekly action plans.

▼ Finally, place some cues in your physical environment to help remind you to practice these pain-management skills. If you practice your program regularly it will work better for you. For example, place notes or stickers where you will see them to remind you to practice a technique. Try putting a star on your mirror, your office or home telephone, or the dashboard of your car. Change the stickers every month or so to help you notice them.

Relaxation Techniques

So much has been said and written about relaxation that most of us are completely confused. It is not a cure-all, but neither is it a hoax. Rather, like most treatment methods, it has specific uses. The advantage of relaxation in the management of arthritis and fibromyalgia is that as muscles become less tense they become easier and less painful to move. In addition to releasing muscle tension throughout the body, relaxation exercises help you to sleep better and feel more refreshed.

Like all exercise, the following techniques require practice in order for you to reap the benefits. If you feel you are not accomplishing anything, be patient and keep trying. Try another method if the one you choose does not seem to work for you. Give each method at least two full weeks for a fair trial. Relaxation techniques should be practiced at least fifteen to twenty minutes a day, five days a week.

With many forms of arthritis and fibromyalgia, it is wise to take short rest periods during the day, to avoid undue fatigue and to relieve stress. This is an excellent time to practice relaxation techniques.

The following are examples of relaxation techniques. When you have chosen the ones that work best for you, you might consider tape-recording the technique. This is not necessary but is sometimes helpful if you find it hard to concentrate. With an inexpensive cassette recorder or CD, you can tape a script or routine to follow so you won't have to look at this book while you are trying to relax. At the end of this chapter you will find information about how to buy relaxation tapes and CDs.

Here are some guidelines that will help you practice the relaxation techniques described in this chapter:

1. Pick a quiet time and place where you will not be disturbed for fifteen to twenty minutes.

2. Try to practice daily, but not less than five times a week.

3. Be patient and don't expect miracles. It will probably take three to four weeks of practice before you really start to notice any benefits.

4. Remember, relaxation should be helpful. At worst, you may find it boring, but if it is unpleasant or makes you nervous, then try other pain-management techniques.

Breathing Exercises

Breathing, especially *diaphragmatic* or *abdominal (belly) breathing,* is a special form of relaxation. In fact, it is an integral part of many of the other techniques described in this chapter. While we all breathe to live, not all of us breathe in the most effective and efficient way. Pain, stress, and tension interfere with our breathing patterns, making each breath shallow rather than deep and relaxing. Therefore, to help us learn to relax, use our lungs to their fullest capacity, and conserve energy, we need to relearn and practice diaphragmatic breathing.

To practice diaphragmatic breathing, find a comfortable position either lying down on your back or sitting in a chair. Relax your shoulders. Next, place one hand on your abdomen just above your navel and below your breastbone, and the other hand on the upper part of your chest. Close your eyes and become aware of your breathing. As you breathe in through your nose, feel your abdomen rising as if it were a balloon filling with air. There should be little movement in your upper chest area. As you breathe out, do so slowly through gently pursed lips and imagine that the balloon is deflating. Once you are able to do the diaphragmatic breathing, you can use it wherever you are to help you relax.

There is another useful breathing exercise called *breath focusing*. It helps us to resist the natural tendency to either hold our breath or breathe shallowly when we anticipate or experience discomfort. When you learn breath focusing, you will find it becomes difficult to hold on to your tension, stress, or pain. Begin by taking a slow, deep breath from your diaphragm. Concentrate on your breathing, breathe in slowly through your nose, hold it for a few seconds, and breathe out through your mouth. As you do this, tell yourself to relax. It is important to concentrate on your breathing, keeping it slow and easy.

Both focused and diaphragmatic breathing help manage your symptoms and also help you deal with other difficult and stressful events.

One problem that people sometimes experience when practicing these breathing exercises is hyperventilation. They tend to breathe too fast or too deeply and have a hard time catching their breath. They may also feel lightheaded, dizzy, or anxious. Hyperventilation is scary but not dangerous. It is caused by having too much oxygen and not enough carbon dioxide in your body. If this happens, stop practicing the technique and breathe normally. If this does not help, breathe into a closed paper bag—not plastic—for a short time. To avoid hyperventilation, keep your breathing slow and easy when practicing these techniques.

Jacobson's Progressive Relaxation

Many years ago a physiologist, Edmund Jacobson, discovered that in order to relax one must know what it feels like to be relaxed and to be tense. He believed that if one could recognize muscle tension, one could then let it go and relax. Thus, he designed a very simple set of exercises to assist with the learning process.*

The first step is to become familiar with the difference between the feeling of tension and the feeling of relaxation. To relax muscles, you need to know how to scan your body, recognize where you are holding tension, and release that tension. This brief exercise will allow you to compare tension and relaxation and, with practice, to spot and release tension anywhere in your body.

Progressive relaxation is best done lying on your back either on a rug or in bed. However, it can be done seated in a comfortable chair. It can even be done while traveling in a car (provided you are not driving at the time), airplane, or train. Choose a quiet time and place where you will not be disturbed for at least fifteen minutes and let go of all outside concerns.

Body Scan

This is an alternative to the Jacobson technique and does not require any movement. Like Jacobson, it is best done on your back, but it can be done in any comfortable position. First, you must become aware of your

---

* Much of this section has been adapted from Gordon Paul, *Insight vs. Desensitization in Psychotherapy: An Experiment in Anxiety Reduction* (Stanford, Calif.: Stanford University Press, 1966).

breathing. Spend a few minutes concentrating on your breath as it enters and leaves your body. Try directing your breath to your belly or abdomen. This is called diaphragmatic breathing and is important for all kinds of relaxation.

After three or four minutes of concentrating on your breathing, move your attention to your toes. Don't move your toes, just think about how they feel. Don't worry if you don't feel anything at all. If you find any tension, let it go as you breathe out.

After a few moments of concentrating on your toes, change your attention to the bottom of your feet. Again, don't move, just concentrate on any sensations you have. Let go of any tension you may find as you breathe out. Next concentrate on the top of your feet and your ankles. After a few more moments shift your attention to your lower legs.

Continue this process, shifting your attention every few moments to another portion of the body, working slowly upward. If you find tension, let it go as you breathe out. If at any time your mind wanders, bring your attention back to the feelings in your body and to your breathing.

This technique can also be used for getting back to sleep, as it helps to clear your mind of worries or other distracting thoughts. The secret is to give full attention to the body scan and don't worry if you fall asleep.

The Relaxation Response

During the early 1970s, Dr. Herbert Benson did extensive work on what he calls the relaxation response. He says that our bodies have several natural states. For example, if you meet a lion on the street, you will probably become quite tense—your response will be a "fight-or-flight" response. After extreme tension, the body's natural response is to relax. This is what happens after a sexual climax. As life becomes more and more complex,

Make yourself as comfortable as possible. Uncross your legs, ankles, and arms. Allow your body to feel completely supported by the surface beneath you.

You may want to close your eyes, as a way of closing out any unnecessary distractions.

Begin by taking a deep breath, breathing in through your nose, filling your chest, and breathing all the way down to the abdomen. When you're ready to breathe out, breathe out through pursed lips slowly and completely. As you breathe out, let as much tension as possible flow out with your breath. Let all your muscles feel heavy, and let your whole body just sink into the surface beneath you.

This exercise will guide you through the major muscle groups, from your feet to your head, asking you first to tense and then to relax those muscles. If you have pain in any part of your body, don't tense that area. Instead just notice any tension that may already be there and let go of that tension.

Become aware of the muscles of your **feet and calves.** Pull your toes up toward your knees. Hold your feet in this position . . . noticing the sensations. . . . Now relax your feet and release the tension. Observe any changes in sensations as you let go of the tension.

Now tighten the large muscles of your **thighs and buttocks.** Hold the muscles tense. And as you do, be aware of the sensations. . . . And now release these muscles, allowing them to feel soft, as if they're melting into the surface beneath you.

Now turn your attention to your **abdomen and chest.** Tense these muscles by holding in your abdomen and tightening the muscles on your chest wall. Notice a tendency to hold your breath as you tense these muscles. Now release the tension. You may feel a natural desire to take a deep breath to release even more of the tension, and so do that now. Breathe in deeply through your nose, and when you breathe out, allow your abdomen and chest to soften.

Now, stretching your fingers out straight, tighten the muscles of your **hands and arms.** Release and feel the tension flowing out and the circulation returning.

Next press your shoulder blades together, tightening the muscles in your **upper back, shoulders, and neck.** This is a place many people carry tension. . . . And relax. You may notice that your muscles feel a little warmer and more alive.

Finally, tighten all the muscles of your **face and head.** Notice the tension around your eyes and in your jaw. Now release the tension, allowing the muscles around your eyes to soften and your mouth to remain slightly open as your jaw relaxes. Notice the difference.

Now take another deep breath, and when you're ready to breathe out, allow any remaining tension to flow out with your breath and your whole body to be even more deeply relaxed.

And now just enjoy this feeling of relaxation for a little while. . . . In this quiet state, notice the heaviness of your muscles . . . and the rhythm of your breathing . . . as you breathe in and breathe out.

Remember this pleasant feeling. You can quiet your mind and body in this way anytime you do this exercise. With practice, you will be able to create this feeling just by taking a deep breath.

As you prepare to end this exercise, picture yourself bringing this feeling of quiet and calm to whatever you are going to do next. And then take one more deep breath and, when you're ready, open your eyes.

our bodies tend to stay in a constant state of tension. Thus, to elicit the relaxation response, many people will consciously need to practice the following exercise, which has four basic elements.

1. **A quiet environment.** To create this, try to tune out or turn off internal stimuli and external distractions.

2. **An object to dwell upon or a mental device.** For example, you might repeat a word or sound like the word *one,* gaze at a symbol like a flower, or concentrate on a feeling such as peace.

3. **A passive attitude.** This is the most essential factor. It is an emptying of all thoughts and distractions from your mind. Thoughts, imagery, and feelings may drift into awareness—don't concentrate on them, just allow them to pass on.

4. **A comfortable position.** You should be comfortable enough to remain in the same position for twenty minutes.

The steps to elicit the relaxation response include:

1. Sit quietly in a comfortable position.

2. Close your eyes.

3. Deeply relax all your muscles, beginning at your feet and progressing up to your face. Keep them relaxed. If you wish, you can use the Body Scan just described.

4. Breathe in through your nose. Become aware of your breathing. As you breathe out through your mouth, say the word *one* silently to yourself. Try to empty all thoughts from your mind; concentrate on *one.*

5. Continue for ten to twenty minutes. You may open your eyes to check the time, but do not use an alarm.

When you finish, sit quietly for several minutes, at first with your eyes closed. Do not stand up for a few minutes.

6. Do not worry about whether you are successful in achieving a deep level of relaxation. Maintain a passive attitude and permit relaxation to occur at its own pace. When distracting thoughts occur, try to ignore them by not dwelling upon them and return to repeating *one*.

7. Practice once or twice daily, but ideally not within two hours after any meal, since digestive processes can interfere with the relaxation response.

You may have noticed that this exercise is similar to meditation. In fact, the relaxation response is based on some of the principles of meditation.

Guided Imagery

Another technique is called guided imagery. This is like a guided daydream where you transport yourself to another time and place. It is as though you were taking a mental stroll. The guided imagery scripts presented on pages 210–213 can be used in several different ways, depending on what technique works best for you. Consider each of the following:

1. Read the script over several times to familiarize yourself with it. Then sit or lie in a quiet place and try to reconstruct the scene in your mind. The script should take ten to fifteen minutes to complete.

2. Have a family member or friend slowly read you the script. Wherever there is a series of dots (. . .), he or she should pause for at least ten seconds.

3. Make a tape or CD of the script and play it to yourself.

A Walk in the Country

You're giving yourself some time to quiet your mind and body. Allow yourself to settle comfortably, wherever you are right now. If you wish, you can close your eyes. Breathe in deeply, through your nose, expanding your abdomen and filling your lungs. Pursing your lips, exhale through your mouth slowly and completely, allowing your body to sink heavily into the surface beneath you. . . . And once again, breathe in through your nose and all the way down to your abdomen and then breathe out slowly through pursed lips—letting go of tension, letting go of anything that's on your mind right now, and just allowing yourself to be present in this moment. . . .

Imagine yourself walking along a peaceful old country road. The sun is warm on your back . . . the birds are singing . . . the air is calm and fragrant.

As you walk along, your mind naturally wanders to the concerns and worries of the day. Then you come upon a box by the side of the road and it occurs to you that this box is a perfect place to leave your cares behind while you enjoy this time in the country. So you open the box and put into it any concerns, worries, or pressures that you're carrying with you. You close the box and fasten it securely, knowing that you can come back and deal with those concerns whenever you're ready.

You feel lighter as you progress down the road. Soon you come across an old gate. The gate creaks as you open it and go through.

You find yourself in an overgrown garden—flowers growing where they've seeded themselves, vines climbing over a fallen tree, soft green wild grasses, and shade trees.

Breathe deeply, smelling the flowers . . . listen to the birds and insects . . . feel the gentle breeze warm against your skin. All of your senses are alive and responding with pleasure to this peaceful time and place.

When you're ready to move on, you leisurely follow a path behind the garden, eventually coming to a more wooded area. As you enter this area, your eyes find the trees and plant life restful to look on. The sun is filtered through the leaves. The air feels mild and a little cooler. You become aware of the sound and fragrance of a nearby stream. You pause and take in the sights and sounds, breathing deeply of the cool and fragrant air several times. . . . And with each breath, you feel more refreshed.

Continuing along the path for a while, you come to the stream. It's clear and clean as it flows and tumbles over the rocks and some fallen logs. You follow the path along the creek for a way, and after a while, you come out into a sunlit clearing, where you discover a small waterfall emptying into a quiet pool of water.

You find a comfortable place to sit for a while, a perfect spot where you can feel completely relaxed.

You feel good as you allow yourself to just enjoy the warmth and solitude of this peaceful place.

After a while, you become aware that it is time to return. You arise and walk back down the path, through the cool and fragrant trees, out into the sun-drenched overgrown garden. . . . One last smell of the flowers and out the creaky gate.

You leave this country retreat for now and return down the road. You notice you feel calm and rested. You know that you can visit this special place whenever you wish to take some time to refresh yourself and renew your energy.

A Walk on the Beach

You're giving yourself some time to quiet your mind and body. Allow yourself to settle comfortably wherever you are right now. If you wish, you can close your eyes. Breathe in deeply through your nose, expanding your abdomen and filling your lungs. And pursing your lips, exhale through your mouth slowly and completely, allowing your body to sink heavily into the surface beneath you. Letting go of tension . . . letting go of anything that's on your mind right now . . . and just allowing yourself to be present in this moment. . . .

Imagine yourself walking along a peaceful white sand beach. . . . The waves are gently lapping on the sand. The birds are singing. The air is calm and fragrant. As you walk along, your mind naturally wanders to the concerns and worries of the day. Then, you come upon a box in the sand and it occurs to you that this box is a perfect place to leave your cares behind while you enjoy this time at the beach.

So you open the box and put into it any concerns, worries, or pressures that you're carrying with you. You close the box and fasten it securely, knowing that you can come back and deal with those concerns whenever you're ready. . . .

You feel lighter as you progress along the beach. Soon, you come across a wooded area. You enter through an opening in the trees. You find yourself in a lovely fern grotto. Wildflowers growing where they've seeded themselves. Vines climbing over a fallen tree. Soft green wild grasses. Shade trees. Breathe deeply, smelling the fragrance of the ocean and the forest . . . Listen to the birds and insects. . . . Feel the gentle breeze warm against your skin . . . All of your senses are alive and responding in pleasure to this peaceful time and place. . . .

When you're ready to move on, you leisurely follow a path, eventually coming to a more wooded area. The air feels mild and a little cooler. You become aware of the sound and fragrance of a nearby stream. You pause, breathing deeply of the cool and fragrant air several times . . . Continuing along the path, you come to the stream. It's clear and clean as it flows and tumbles over the rocks and some fallen logs. . . .

You follow the path along the creek for a way, and after a while, you come out into a sunlit clearing where you discover a small waterfall emptying into a quiet pool of water . . . You find a comfortable place to sit for a time. A perfect niche where you can feel completely relaxed. You feel good as you allow yourself to just enjoy the warmth and solitude of this peaceful place. . . .

After a while, you become aware that it's time to return . . . You walk back down the path through the cool and fragrant trees, out into the fern grotto, one last smell of the forest and out to the beach. . . .

You leave this retreat for now and return down the beach, noticing that you feel calm and rested. You know that you can visit this special place whenever you wish to take some time to refresh yourself and renew your energy.

When you are ready to return, take a deep breath and open your eyes.

Vivid Imagery

This is a little like guided imagery but can be used for longer periods or while you are engaged in other activities.

One way to use imagery is to recall pleasant scenes from your past. For example, try to remember every detail of a special holiday or party or vacation that made you happy. Who was there? What happened? What did you talk about? Another way to use imagery is to fill in the details of a pleasant fantasy. How would you spend a million dollars? What would be your ideal romantic encounter? What would your ideal home or garden be like?

Sometimes warm imagery can be especially helpful, such as thinking of yourself on a warm beach or visiting a tropical island. On the other hand, if you live somewhere that is very warm, cool imagery such as a forest or shaded path may be more relaxing.

Another form of vivid imagery is to think of symbols that represent painful parts of your body. For example, a painful joint might be red or might have a tight band around it or even a lion biting it.

Now try to change the image. Make the red fade until there is no color left, or imagine the band stretching and stretching until it falls off. Change the lion into a purring kitten.

A final way to use vivid imagery is to help you with goal setting (see Chapter 6). After you set your weekly action plan, spend a few minutes imagining yourself taking a walk, doing your exercises, or taking your medications. Studies have shown that these few minutes of imagery will help you accomplish your goal. Many people become very skilled at vivid imagery. They find that as they change their pain images, the pain decreases.

Distraction

The distraction technique, also referred to as attention refocusing, is especially helpful to use during short activities that you know are painful or troublesome, such as climbing stairs or doing certain chores. It is also useful when you are having difficulty falling asleep or returning to sleep. Distraction works by deliberately changing the focus of your mind's attention. It is difficult for the mind to focus well on more than one thing at a time; therefore, by refocusing your mind's attention on something other than the pain, discomfort, or worries that interfere with sleep, you diminish these symptoms.

The following are some examples of how you can use your mind to distract yourself from your symptoms.

▼ While climbing stairs, plan exactly what you will be doing when you get to the top. Be as detailed as possible. Or you might name a different bird or flower for each step. You can even try to visualize a bird or flower for every letter of the alphabet.

▼ During any painful activity, think of a person's name, a bird, a food, or whatever, for every letter of the alphabet. If you get stuck on one letter, go on to the next. (This is also a good exercise if you have problems sleeping.)

▼ While sweeping, vacuuming, or mopping, imagine that the floor is a map of North America. Try to name all the states and provinces going from east to west or north to south. You can also do this with the map of Europe or, if you are really good in geography, Africa. If geography is not your strong suit, think of the floor as your favorite store and locate each department.

▼ When getting up from a chair or out of a car, imagine that you are in a spaceship where you are almost weightless, floating effortlessly upward. Or try counting backward from one thousand by threes, each time getting as far as you can until you are standing. Try to break your old record.

▼ While opening a jar, think of as many uses as you can for the jar. Or try to remember the words of a song and imagine the story taking place inside the jar.

There are, of course, a million variations as to how you can refocus your mind's attention away from the pain and onto something else. These are examples of short-term distraction techniques. Distraction also works well for longer activities or projects or when the pain tends to last longer. In these cases, the mind is not focused internally, but rather externally on some type of activity. For example, if you have continual pain or are feeling slightly depressed, find an activity that interests and distracts you from the problem. The activity can be almost anything–gardening, cooking, reading, going to a movie, or doing volunteer work. A mark of a successful self-manager is that he or she has a variety of interests and always seems to be doing something.

Mindfulness Meditation

There are many types of meditation. In fact, meditation is a part of most, if not every, religious or spiritual tradition. The purpose of meditation is to quiet the mind. It may also help the individual to quiet the body. For this reason, meditation is often a useful technique for managing stress and other symptoms such as pain, fatigue, or shortness of breath. Mindfulness meditation is one type of meditation that can be practiced by anyone. All that you need to begin is a quiet place and five or more minutes. Start by sitting in a chair with your feet flat on the floor and your hands in your lap or on your knees. If you wish and are able to, you can sit on the floor with crossed legs or in a more traditional yoga position. How you sit, however, does not matter.

The essence of mindfulness meditation is to concentrate fully on your breathing. It is best if you can do diaphragmatic or belly breathing, but you do not have to take deep breaths. It is important to keep your full attention on your breathing. Breathe in slowly; hold the breath for a moment, then breathe out slowly. At all times, concentrate on your breathing.

While this seems fairly simple, you will soon find that your mind easily wanders. This is called "having a monkey mind." As soon as you notice that your mind is wandering, bring your attention back to your breathing. At first you may not be able to attend to your breathing for more than a minute or two. You will improve, however, with practice.

When you are doing this type of meditation, you may become very aware of your body. For example, your eye may itch or you may become uncomfortable in your sitting position. When this happens, first do nothing but pay attention to your breathing. In many cases you will find that the discomfort goes away. If it continues, however, scratch the itch or change your position. As you do this, pay full attention to what you are doing. With mindfulness meditation it is important to be fully aware of what you are doing at that moment!

Like all other self-management techniques, mindfulness meditation requires practice. You will not get results immediately; however, if you practice this for fifteen to thirty minutes a day, four or five times a week, you will find over time that this can be a great pain management tool.

Prayer

Over the years, we have had many people tell us that prayer has been very helpful in managing their pain. In many ways, prayer is similar to some relaxation techniques, and in other ways, it may be a distraction technique. However, one does not need to have a scientific rationale for everything. As the oldest of all pain-management techniques, prayer is very important for many successful arthritis pain managers.

Self-Talk: "I Know I Can"

All of us talk to ourselves all the time. For example, when waking up in the morning, we think, "I really don't want to get out of bed. I'm tired and don't want to go to work today." Or at the end of an enjoyable evening we think, "Gee, that was really fun. I should get out more often." These habitual things we think or say to ourselves are referred to as "self-talk."

All of our self-talk is learned from others and becomes a part of us as we grow up. It comes in many forms, mostly negative. Negative self-statements are usually in the form of phrases that begin like these: "I just can't do . . . ," "If only I could or didn't . . . ," "I just don't have the energy. . . ." This type of self-talk reflects the doubts and fears we have about ourselves in general and about our abilities to deal with arthritis and its symptoms in particular. In fact, negative self-talk can worsen pain, depression, and fatigue.

What we say to ourselves plays a major role in determining our success or failure in becoming good self-managers. Therefore, learning to make self-talk work *for* you instead of *against* you, by changing or replacing those negative statements with positive ones, will help you manage your symptoms more effectively. This change, as with any habit, requires practice. It includes the following steps:

1. **Listen carefully to what you say to or about yourself,** both out loud and silently. Then write down all the negative self-talk statements. Pay special attention to the things you say during times that are particularly difficult or stressful for you. For example, what do you say to yourself when getting up in the morning with pain, while doing those exercises you don't really like, when feeling blue, or when faced with problematic situations?

2. **Work on replacing each negative statement** you identified with a positive one, and write these down. Positive statements should reflect the better you, and your decision to be in control. For example, negative statements such as "I don't want to get up," "I'm too tired, and I hurt," "I can't do the things I like anymore so why bother," or "I'm good for nothing," become positive messages, such as "I have the energy to get up and do the things I enjoy," or "I know I can do anything I believe I can," "People like me, and I feel good about myself," or "Other people need and depend on me; I'm worthwhile."

3. **Read and rehearse these positive statements,** mentally or with another person. It is this conscious repetition or memorization of the positive statements that will help you replace those old, habitual negative statements.

4. **Practice these new statements in real situations.** This practice, along with time and patience, will help the new patterns of thinking become automatic.

Once established, positive self-talk can be a powerful self-management tool that can help you cope better with specific symptoms, as well as master some of the other skills discussed in this book.

As with exercise and other acquired skills, using your mind to manage your condition requires both practice and time before you'll begin to notice the benefits. Therefore, if you feel like you are not accomplishing anything, don't give up. Be patient and keep on trying.

Heat and Cold

The use of heat and cold are effective and inexpensive ways to achieve temporary relief of muscle and joint pain.

Heat is most effective for reducing the pain associated with muscle tension and stiffness, and when there is little or no inflammation. It works by increasing the blood flow to the skin and muscles around the painful area. This, in turn, enhances muscle nutrition and relaxation. When the muscles relax, pain and stiffness decrease. Some easy ways to apply heat locally to an area of the body include a heating pad, hot water bottle, hot towels, hot packs, or a heating lamp. Warm baths, showers, a hot tub, sauna, or an electric mattress pad are good ways to help soothe the whole body; these methods may be particularly beneficial for the person with fibromyalgia.

You can make a hot pack by filling a sock or other cloth bag with a grain like rice or barley (not cooked). Put this in the microwave for 2–3 minutes to warm. Always test the temperature to make sure it is not too hot. Do not use popcorn!

For some people, applying cold may work better. Applying ice helps to stop muscle spasms and numbs the nerves that are sending pain signals. Ice also reduces the blood flow to the painful area, which works to reduce inflammation and swelling. Some quick and easy ways to apply ice include the use of large bags of frozen peas or corn, plastic storage bags filled with ice cubes, or the ice bags or packs that can be purchased at the store. When using any type of ice pack, it is important to wrap it in a wet towel or cloth to avoid skin burns from the cold. In fact, whether you are using heat or cold, do not apply it for longer than fifteen to twenty minutes.

Other methods of warming and cooling a painful area include the use of topical creams or liniments. Many of these products contain menthol or alcohol and camphor, which affect the skin first by warming it, then cooling it. These products should not be used with other applications of heat or cold, such as heating pads or ice.

Massage

Many people find that massage or rubbing the painful area can be very helpful. Massage is actually one of the oldest forms of pain management for arthritis. Hippocrates (c. 460–380 B.C.) said that "physicians must be experienced in many things, but assuredly also in rubbing that can bind a joint that is loose and loosen a joint that is too hard." Self-massage is a simple procedure that involves the use of applied pressure and stretching to an area of the body. It can be performed with little practice or preparation. When done correctly, massage can be very beneficial for both mind and body. Not only does it relax tense muscles, but it also improves movement and stimulates the blood flow and nutrition to the skin, underlying tissues, and muscles.

The following are some basic massage techniques. A little experience with each will help you decide which works best for you.

Also remember to allow yourself a minute to relax and let the tension subside after you do the self-massage. Try some deep breathing in combination with the massage to help produce even better results.

Stroking

Fit your hand to the contour of the muscle you want to massage and move it over the skin along the length of the muscle. By slightly cupping the hand, the palm and fingers will glide firmly over the muscle. A slow rhythmic movement repeated over the tense or sore area works best. Experiment with different pressures.

Kneading

If you have ever reached up and squeezed your tense neck or shoulder muscles, you were kneading. Grasp the muscle between the palm and fingers or between the thumb and fingers (as if you are kneading dough), then slightly lift and squeeze it. Don't pinch the skin, but work deeply into the muscle itself. A slow, rhythmic squeeze and release works best. Don't knead one spot for more than fifteen or twenty seconds.

Deep Circular Movement or Friction

To create friction that penetrates into the muscle, make small circular movements with the tips of the fingers, the thumb, or the heel of the hand, depending on how large an area you want to massage. Keep the fingers, thumb, or heel in one place, and begin lightly making small circles. Slowly increase the pressure, but don't overdo it. After ten seconds or so, move to another spot and repeat the movement.

Self-massage is particularly useful in helping to relieve pain and muscle tension in localized areas of the body that are easy to reach. Sometimes, however, it is difficult to relax completely and effectively when also trying to massage your back, neck, or shoulders. Therefore, consider some alternatives, such as finding someone else to massage those areas or buying a handheld massager. If you cannot afford to buy an electric massager, you might try making your own. Put a tennis ball in a sock or stocking, then by moving the sock up or down, you can place it in the area you want to massage. When you've got the spot, move to roll the ball between your back and a wall or the back of a chair. Try it and you will see it is much easier than it sounds.

It is important to note that there are times when massage is not appropriate to use: for example, on a "hot joint," an infected joint, or when there is phlebitis, thrombophlebitis, or skin sores or rashes.

A Word of Caution

The pain-management techniques taught in this chapter, along with other techniques such as self-hypnosis, biofeedback, and acupressure, are still being studied for their usefulness in managing arthritis. We make no special claims for them. Many people in our classes report substantial benefits from these practices, and we feel that they have merit if used as an adjunct to, and not a substitute for, a basic, sound program that is medically directed.

Hypnosis is generally not recommended for people with arthritis. Like certain narcotics, it can mask pain and may thereby cause you to damage your joints. Some of the techniques discussed in this chapter are similar to those used in *self*-hypnosis, however.

Unfortunately, various pain-management techniques are sold in expensive packages as cure-alls. Such expensive courses and treatments are *not* necessary. If you want to further explore these techniques, check the following points first to avoid unnecessary expense and disappointment.

1. Is the course or treatment offered by a reputable institution?

2. Is the cost reasonable?

3. Are claims or promises made for a cure? If so, look elsewhere.

Chapter 15

Getting a Good Night's Sleep

Sleep is vital for maintaining a healthy outlook on life. It allows our bodies to heal and our energy to be replenished. As explained in Chapter 5, lack of restful sleep also contributes to fibromyalgia.

Beds

A comfortable bed that allows ease of movement and good body support is the first requirement for a good night's sleep. This usually means a good-quality, firm mattress that supports the spine and does not allow the body to sag in the middle of the bed. A bed board, made of three-quarter-inch or half-inch (1 or 2 cm) plywood, can be placed between the mattress and the box spring to increase firmness. Bedboards can be bought commercially or constructed at home.

Heated waterbeds or airbeds are helpful for some people with arthritis because they support weight evenly by conforming to the body's shape. Others find these beds uncomfortable. If you are interested, try one out at a friend's home or a hotel for a few nights to decide if it is right for you.

An electric blanket or mattress pad, used at a low heat, is another effective way of providing heat while sleeping, especially for cool or damp nights. Or you might try a wool mattress pad. If you decide to use one or the other, be sure to follow the instructions carefully.

Sleeping Positions

The best sleeping position depends on which joints are involved. For most people without arthritis of the knees or hips, the best position is sleeping on one's side or back. In either case, it is best to use a small, soft pillow to support the curvature of the neck and maintain normal neck alignment. Pillows may also be used under the knees to relieve back pain. However, care should be taken not to maintain this position continuously. If you have knee problems, check with your doctor before using a pillow under your knees even for a short period, as it can cause knee contractures. In the side-lying position, a small pillow can be placed between the knees.

For people with hip or knee problems, the best sleeping position is one where the knees are straight and the hips are in a neutral position (not rotated to the sides). There are also a few dos and don'ts.

▼ Do try to rest on your stomach for ten or fifteen minutes a day. This will help prevent flexion contractures of the hips.

▼ If it does not bother you, try putting a small pillow under your ankles while sleeping on your back. (This will keep your knees straight.)

▼ Don't sleep with pillows under your knees, even if this is more comfortable.

For people with back problems, often a comfortable way to sleep is in the side-lying position with knees bent. In this position, it can be helpful to place a pillow between the knees to alleviate stress on the hips and lower back. A pillow can also be placed under the upper arm to reduce stress on the shoulder joint. But in most cases, your body will tell you the best position. There is no single right way.

If you have ankylosing spondylitis, there are some specific sleep positions that will help prevent deformity and loss of mobility of the spine. Sleep on your stomach or flat on your back. Avoid using high pillows under your head; sleep without a pillow if possible. Place a small pillow between your shoulder blades when you sleep on your back.

Sleeping Pills

Sedatives and sleeping pills should be used with caution. They may be habit-forming, suppress important stages of sleep, and cause depression. They only rarely solve sleep problems; the medication taken to control sleep may actually produce a disturbed night's sleep. (This is also true of alcohol.) If you are using medications and decide to stop, do so gradually. You should also know that you may have restless sleep for a night or two after stopping sleeping pills. Don't get discouraged and go back on pills. Normal sleep will return in a few nights.

Certain types of antidepressant medications can be helpful for sleep that is disturbed by pain and also for treating fibromyalgia. The dosage used is much smaller than that used for depression. These medications do not have the potential addictive side effects that many sedatives and sleeping pills have. Ask your physician about them.

Insomnia

There is no known serious medical complication from lack of sleep. If you go without sleep long enough, you will fall asleep, so don't worry. If you can't sleep, don't lie in bed feeling guilty or bored—get up and do something you enjoy, like reading a book or listening to music, until you are sleepy. You need less sleep as you age, so be sure your insomnia is not due to sleeping too much.

Still, insomnia is a problem that affects all of us at one time or another. It can be a cause of concern if it occurs frequently and involves recurrent daytime fatigue or depression. The causes of insomnia are many, some of which are feelings of anxiety or worry, pain or discomfort due to a medical condition, or an unfamiliar sleeping environment. Other contributing factors may be improper self-treatment or failure to follow the practitioner's recommended dosage or directions for medications. If your sleeping problem continues, you may want to seek a physician's advice.

Some hints for a more comfortable night's sleep include the following:

▼ Maintain a regular sleep schedule so that you go to bed and awaken at about the same time each night and morning.

▼ For relief of pain and inflammation at night, take aspirin or anti-inflammatory drugs as your doctor prescribes and be sure to take the proper dose at bedtime. Painkillers should be used with great caution. To maintain a good level of aspirin or anti-inflammatory drugs throughout the night, try timed-release aspirin (available by prescription). If pain without inflammation is a problem, Tylenol also comes in a timed-release form.

▼ Use some of the relaxation techniques described in Chapter 14, or create one of your own that is particularly relaxing to you and will settle the day's thoughts and ease the body's tensions. (Distracting yourself by counting backward from one thousand by twos or threes is especially helpful.)

▼ Wait until you are sleepy and your body is ready and eager to go to sleep; going to bed early to ensure a good night's sleep is often counterproductive.

▼ Avoid caffeine (coffee, tea, soft drinks, chocolate) for several hours before bedtime because it can act as a stimulant.

▼ Moderate your alcohol intake; alcohol may cause an erratic night's sleep and restlessness. Avoid any alcohol for three or four hours before bedtime.

▼ Provide yourself with a comfortable environment. Your environment includes mattress, lighting, noise level, temperature, and ventilation.

▼ Try taking a warm bath (not hot) before going to bed.

▼ Get as much exercise as you can during the day, but refrain from exercising immediately before bedtime.

▼ Don't do things that excite you just before going to sleep.

▼ Avoid naps if you are having problems sleeping at night.

▼ Get used to doing the same things every night before going to bed. By developing a "time-to-get-ready-for-bed" routine, you will be telling your body that it's time to start winding down and relaxing.

▼ Ask your doctor about tricyclic antidepressants to enhance deep sleep cycles. This is particularly helpful for fibromyalgia.

If you do wake up with stiffness during the night, try some easier exercises (or small amounts of exercise in the pain-free range) right in the bed to reduce discomfort and pain, allowing for a more undisturbed and restful sleep.

Do You Sleep "Like a Baby"?

If you fall asleep as soon as your "head hits the pillow" or regularly fall asleep in front of the TV, and yet you are tired when you wake up in the morning in spite of a full night's sleep, you may have a sleep disorder. People who have the most common sleep disorder, obstructive sleep apnea, often don't know it. When they are asked about their sleep, they respond, "I sleep just fine." Sleep specialists believe that obstructive sleep apnea is very common and alarmingly underdiagnosed.

With sleep apnea, the soft tissue in the throat or nose relaxes during sleep and blocks the airway, causing extreme effort to breathe. The person struggles against the blockage for up to a minute, then wakes just long enough to gasp air, falling back asleep to start the cycle all over again, never aware that he or she has awakened dozens of times per night. Getting the deep sleep needed to restore the daily toll on our muscles and joints is never achieved, leading to more pain and fatigue for someone with arthritis or fibromyalgia.

Sleep apnea is a serious medical problem, even life-threatening. Sleep apnea has been linked to heart disease and stroke and is believed to be a cause of death for many who die in their sleep from a heart attack. Sleep experts suggest that people who are tired all the time in spite of a full night's sleep or who find they need more sleep now than when they were younger should be evaluated for sleep apnea or other sleep disorders, especially if they (or their spouse) report snoring. For people with arthritis or fibromyalgia, getting help for a sleep disorder can make a real difference in pain.

Chapter 16

Depression, Fatigue, and Other Symptoms

Sometimes people with arthritis suffer from other problems brought on by their pain, by frustration, or even by the arthritis medications they take. These problems, or people's common response to them, can make life much worse than the arthritis alone. In this chapter we deal with several such symptoms, some of which you might not even recognize as being related to arthritis. This chapter covers depression, pain, fatigue, and constipation.

Depression

One of the most frequent symptoms associated with arthritis is depression. (Some people prefer to say they are "unhappy," "blue," or "feeling down" instead of "depressed.") Depression, pain, and concerns about growing older are often parts of a vicious circle. The more depressed you are, the more pain you feel; the more pain you feel, the more stressed you become; the more stressed you become, the more depressed you are. Depression makes you tired, fatigue aggravates your depression and pain, and so on.

We have already discussed a number of ways to deal with pain, including heat, relaxation, and exercise. Continue to do these things when you are feeling well in order to maintain your good spirits. And take your med-

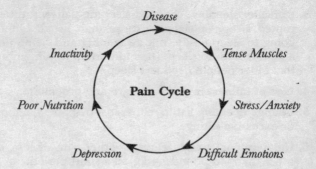

icine and do your exercises—even if you don't feel like it. When you are feeling down, it is especially important to pay attention to maintaining these techniques. Besides your regular self-management techniques, however, you also want to take steps to lick the depression that is making everything worse.

It is easy to tell when you have pain. But it is not as easy to recognize when you are depressed. Just as there are many degrees of pain, there are also many different degrees of depression. If your arthritis is a significant problem, you almost certainly have or have had some problems with depression; such problems are normal. Everyone feels depressed at some time. The following fourteen signs have to do with depression, and you probably have had some of them, in either mild or severe form.

1. **Loss of interest in friends or activities.** Not being home to friends, perhaps not even answering the doorbell or the telephone.

2. **Isolation.** Not wanting to talk to anyone, avoiding friends you happen to meet in the street.

3. **Difficulty sleeping,** changed sleeping patterns, interrupted sleep, or sleeping more than usual. Often, going to sleep easily, but awakening and being unable to return to sleep. (It is important to remember that older people need less sleep.)

4. **Loss of interest in personal care and grooming.**

5. **Change in eating habits,** either loss of interest in food or excessive eating.

6. **Unintentional weight change,** either gain or loss, of more than ten pounds (4 kg) in a short period.

7. **A general feeling of unhappiness lasting longer than six weeks.**

8. **Loss of interest in being held or in sex.** Intimacy problems can sometimes be due to medications, and they are very important, so be sure to talk them over with your doctor.

9. **Suicidal thoughts.**

10. **Frequent accidents.** Watch for a pattern of increased carelessness, accidents while walking or driving, dropping things, and so forth.

11. **Low self-image.** A feeling of worthlessness, a negative image of your body, wondering if it is all worth it.

12. **Frequent arguments, anger, and hostility.** A tendency to blow up easily over minor matters, over things that never bothered you before. This is how some people express depression.

13. **Loss of energy.** Feeling tired all the time.

14. **Feeling confused and unable to concentrate.** Inability to make decisions.

If some of these seem familiar, you may well be depressed. There are more than a dozen things you can do to change the situation. But since you are depressed, you may not feel like making the effort. Force yourself or get someone to help you into action. Find someone to talk with. Here are fourteen actions:

1. **Get help.** If your unhappiness has caused you to think seriously about killing yourself, get help. Call on your doctor, good friends, a member of the clergy, a psychologist, or a social worker. Call your mental health center, doctor, suicide prevention center, a friend, clerical counselor, or senior center. Do not delay. These feelings will pass and you will feel better. Even if you do not feel like hurting yourself, counseling may help you get on with a happier life. Getting help is not a sign of weakness; it is a sign of strength.

2. **Review your medications.** Are you taking tranquilizers or narcotic painkillers? These include drugs such as Valium, Librium, reserpine, codeine, vicodin, sleeping medications, and other "downers." These drugs intensify depression, and the sooner you can stop taking them, the better off you will be. Your depression may well be a drug side effect. If you are not sure what you are taking or what the side effects might be, check with the doctor or pharmacist. Before discontinuing a prescription medication, always check, at least by phone, with the prescribing physician, as there may be important reasons for continuing its use or there may be withdrawal reactions.

3. **Moderate alcohol consumption.** Are you drinking alcohol in order to feel better? Alcohol is also a downer. There is virtually no way to escape depression unless you free your brain of these chemicals. For most people, one or two drinks in the evening is not

a problem, but if your mind is not free of alcohol during most of the day, you are having trouble with this drug.

4. **Continue your daily activities.** Get dressed every day, make your bed, get out of the house, go shopping, walk your dog. Plan and cook meals. Force yourself to do these things even if you don't feel like it.

5. **Visit with friends.** Call them on the phone, plan to go to the movies or on other outings.

6. **Join a group.** Get involved in a church group, a discussion group at a senior citizen club, a community college class, a self-help class, or a senior nutrition program.

7. **Make plans and carry them out.** Look to the future. Plan a future social event or trip. Plant some young trees. Look forward to your grandchildren's graduation from college, even if they are in kindergarten.

8. **Don't move to a new setting without first visiting for a few weeks.** Moving can be a sign of withdrawal, and depression often intensifies when you are in a location away from friends and acquaintances. Your troubles may move with you.

9. **Take a vacation with relatives or friends.** Vacations can be as simple as a few days in a nearby city or a resort just a few miles down the road. Rather than go alone, look into trips sponsored by colleges, senior centers, or church groups.

10. **Do twenty to thirty minutes of physical exercise every day.** Exercise can be a very potent treatment.

11. **Make a list of self-rewards.** Take care of yourself. You can reward yourself by reading at a set time, seeing a special play, or by anything big or small that you can look forward to.

12. **Get a pet.** Animals are wonderful, cheerful companions.

13. **Use positive self-talk** (see page 218).

14. **Help someone else.** Volunteer.

Depression feeds on depression, so break the cycle. The success of everything else in this book depends on it. Depression is not permanent, and you can hasten its disappearance. Focus on your pride, your friends, your future goals, your positive surroundings. How you respond to depression is a self-fulfilling prophecy. When you believe that things will get better, they will. Positive self-talk, used often, can help you believe.

Finally, if you are unable to get out of your depression despite your best efforts, talk to your doctor. A short course of antidepressant medication, counseling, or both may be needed to get you back to your old self.

Pain

Although we have talked a lot about pain in earlier chapters, here we would like to review some basic principles and discuss the connection between pain and mood.

1. **Keep active when you have pain.** Get dressed in your favorite clothes. Women, put on makeup. Men, shave. Now do something. Go to work, go out shopping, go to a movie. All of these activities will make you look and feel good, and they will help keep your mind off the pain. If instead you stay home in your favorite robe, stay in bed, or mope around the house, you will have too much time to think about your pain, and it will seem worse than it is.

2. **Exercise.** Unless you are in a "flare" and have "hot" joints, exercise will help. Some of the pain of arthritis is due to stiff, unused muscles. Therefore, it is very

important to keep your muscles in strong, supple condition. Muscle strength will also help keep your joints stable. See chapters 9, 10, 11, and 12.

3. **Practice relaxation exercises.** Relaxed muscles and nerve endings send out fewer pain messages, and thus you have less pain. See Chapter 14.

4. **Don't be a martyr.** Pain is individual, and it cannot be seen. Therefore, don't be afraid to tell friends and family members that you are in pain. Ask for help in carrying groceries, making beds, or mowing the lawn. Remember that people usually can't see your arthritis or tell that it is hurting you. A direct request for help is not being dependent; it is a direct, honest, and often necessary communication. Besides, you are giving your friends a gift by allowing them to help you.

5. **Understand that pain and mood are related.** Pain is closely related to stress and depression. Reducing stress and depression will also reduce pain. Sometimes people are not aware of how closely attitude and pain are related. We suggest a simple exercise. For a week, keep a Pain/Mood Diary. Each day, put a dot somewhere between "No Pain" and "Terrible Pain" to indicate your pain for that day. Do the same for your mood. After a week, connect all the pain marks and all the mood marks. You may be surprised to see the connections between your mood and your pain.

Fatigue

There is no question about it, arthritis can drain your energy. This is particularly true of rheumatoid arthritis and fibromyalgia. But fatigue can be a problem in any type of arthritis.

Activities are more energy-demanding when you have arthritis, especially an inflammatory type. The body is less efficient in its use of energy reserved for everyday activities, in part because some of this energy is used in the body's attempt to heal itself.

Fatigue can have many causes, such as the following:

▼ **Inactivity.** Muscles not used become deconditioned; that is, they become less efficient in doing what they are supposed to do. The heart, which is made of muscular tissue, can also become deconditioned. When this happens, the heart's ability to pump blood and necessary nutrients and oxygen to other parts of the body is decreased. When muscles do not receive nutrients and oxygen necessary to function properly, they tire more easily than muscles in good condition.

▼ **Poor nutrition.** Food is our basic source of energy. If the fuel we take in is not of top quality and in proper quantities, fatigue can result. For some people, obesity results in fatigue. Extra weight increases the amount of energy needed to perform daily activities and adds stress to joints. For others, being underweight can cause problems associated with fatigue. More about nutrition can be found in Chapter 13.

▼ **Insufficient or poor-quality rest.** For a variety of reasons, there are times when we do not get enough sleep or have poor-quality sleep. You may also have a sleep disorder and not know it. See "Do You Sleep Like a Baby?" in Chapter 15.

▼ **Emotions.** Stress and depression can also cause significant fatigue. Most people are aware of the connection between stress and feeling tired, but fatigue is also an important symptom of depression.

▼ **Medication side effects.** Check with your doctor about this.

▼ **Underactive thyroid.** Again, ask your doctor about this.

If fatigue is a problem for you, your first job is to *determine the cause*. Are you eating well? Are you exercising? Are you getting enough good-quality sleep? If you answer no to any of these questions, you may be on your way to determining one or more of the reasons for your fatigue.

The important thing to remember about your fatigue is that it may be caused by many things other than your arthritis. Therefore, in order to fight and prevent fatigue, you must address the cause of your fatigue.

People often say they can't exercise because they feel fatigued. This creates a vicious cycle: People are fatigued because of a lack of exercise, yet they don't exercise because of the fatigue. If this is your problem, then, believe it or not, motivating yourself to do a little exercise next time you are fatigued may be the answer. You don't have to run a marathon. Just go outdoors and take a short walk. If this is not possible, then walk around your house. See Chapter 9 for more information on getting started on an exercise program.

If emotions are causing your fatigue, rest will not help. In fact, it may make you feel worse. Fatigue is often a sign of depression.

If your fatigue is caused by your disease, then there are several things you can do.

1. Conserve your energy (see Chapter 7).

2. Do the obvious—rest! Take a short nap once or twice a day. If this is impossible, then just relax. Try doing a relaxation exercise (see page 206).

3. Fatigue, like pain and fear, cannot be seen and is not understood by most people. Therefore, tell your boss, friends, and family that fatigue is one of the

problems of your arthritis and that you may have to take short rests from time to time. Most employers are more than willing to allow a little extra rest time for good employees. You, your family, your friends, and your employer should understand that there is a difference between fatigue and being lazy.

4. Take a good long look at yourself. Will you allow yourself to rest? Many of us build our self-image around the ideal of being indestructible—supermom, macho man, or the perfect worker. If this is you, then reassess your position. Fatigue is one of the body's major early warning systems; it is telling you to take heed. Tune in to your own body and follow its directions.

Constipation

Constipation is common among people with arthritis. One reason for this is that many people with arthritis are not as physically active as they once were. Another is that a number of arthritis medications tend to be constipating.

To prevent or deal with constipation, keep these suggestions in mind:

1. **Pay attention to your body's signals.** If you feel you need to go to the bathroom, don't wait. Go. It is easier for your body to develop its own natural schedule for bowel movements when you pay attention to the warning signals.

2. **Take your time in the bathroom.**

    ▼ Take deep breaths to relax the muscles.

    ▼ Don't strain.

    ▼ To make sure you take your time, have something to read or a radio in your bathroom.

3. **Don't force your body into a rigid schedule.** There is no need to have a bowel movement every day.

4. **Don't overuse laxatives.** If you don't feel pain or discomfort when you go to the bathroom, don't take laxatives to force yourself onto a different schedule.

   Laxatives can make minor problems with constipation more persistent. If you use one frequently, your intestines can become dependent on it, with the result that you become constipated when you stop the laxative. If this happens, don't try to solve the problem by going back to the laxative. Instead, give your system time to adjust to functioning on its own. Help it along by following the other suggestions in this section.

   If you must use a laxative, use one based on psyllium (Metamucil, Hydrocil Instant, Fiberall, Serutan). Psyllium is a natural product that holds water and adds bulk. When using one of these products be sure to drink plenty of water or other fluid (six to eight glasses a day).

   In general, try to avoid antacids; many can be constipating. If you must take an antacid while constipated, choose one that tends not to be constipating. Avoid milk of magnesia. (Maalox, Mylanta, and Gelusil are possible substitutes.) You can now buy "stool softeners" over the counter. Ask your pharmacist about these.

5. **Manage your stress level.** Organize your work schedule to minimize your efforts and maximize your strength. For example, do all the upstairs work at one time, all downstairs work another time. Take rest periods. Also, try out the relaxation techniques discussed in Chapter 14.

6. **Eat slowly.** Mealtime should be a period of rest. When you eat, sit down, concentrate on eating, and

try to enjoy your food. Don't think about problems or things you have to do. Chew slowly and thoroughly.

7. **Drink plenty of fluids.** Water adds bulk to the stool. This keeps the stool soft and makes it easier for your muscles to move it through your intestinal tract. Try to drink at least two quarts or liters of fluids each day—about eight glasses. Plain water is good (warm or cool) but mineral water, club soda, coffee, tea, juice, milk, and soup also count (although caffeine can dehydrate).

8. **Exercise.** Physical activity will help your body eliminate waste more smoothly and easily.

9. **Eat prunes or drink prune juice.** Prunes and prune juice naturally contain a chemical substance that eases constipation. (If you are trying to lose weight, keep in mind that prune juice has more calories than most juices.)

10. **Gradually add fiber to your diet.** Our bodies cannot digest certain parts of most fruits, vegetables, and whole-grain products. The parts we cannot digest are referred to as fiber. Fiber is a natural laxative. It holds water in and adds bulk to the stool, which makes it softer and easier to expel. Fiber also helps waste pass through the lower intestine more quickly.

You can increase the amount of fiber (including insoluble fiber) in your diet by eating more fruits and vegetables and more whole-grain breads, cereals, and crackers. Both cooked and raw vegetables and fruits provide significant amounts of fiber. Whole-wheat bread is a good source of insoluble fiber, as are whole-grain cereals made from wheat. Wheat bran and bran cereal are excellent sources of insoluble fiber, but should always be eaten in small quantities with plenty of fluids. If dry cereals or wheat bran seem to irritate your system, try hot cereals instead.

Be sure to add fiber to your diet gradually over weeks or months. If you don't, you may overwhelm your digestive system, experience problems with gas, and become very uncomfortable.

Part VI

Your Medical Resources

Chapter 17

Working with Your Doctor: A Joint Venture

Choosing a Doctor

There are many different kinds of doctors, and sometimes it is difficult to know which kind to work with for what. Fortunately, most people with arthritis do not need a specialist on a regular basis. Therefore, it often is best to find a doctor who can help you with all of your health problems. For most, this will be either an *internist* or a *family practitioner*.

An internist has had special training in the care of adults. Internists take care of all common adult health problems, including arthritis. A family practitioner has special training in taking care of all the common health problems that occur in a family. Thus, a family practitioner may assist at the birth of a baby and also take care of grandmother's arthritis. As a rule, the fewer doctors you have, the better coordinated your health care will be.

For people with difficult arthritis, a *rheumatologist* can be a big help. Rheumatologists are internists with additional training in arthritis and rheumatic diseases. If your arthritis is resistant to treatment or if you have an inflammatory arthritis such as psoriatic arthritis, systemic lupus, or juvenile arthritis, seek out a rheumatologist.

A special note of thanks to David Sobel, M.D., for his assistance with this chapter.

Most important, if you have rheumatoid arthritis, we strongly advise that you see a rheumatologist as early as possible and periodically thereafter. As we noted in Chapter 2, rheumatoid arthritis is almost always best managed by early and continued use of some of the newer drugs. Rheumatologists are the doctors most familiar with these drugs and are most comfortable with their early use; other doctors tend to use them too little, too late.

To find a rheumatologist, look in your telephone directory or ask your doctor if he or she thinks a referral might be appropriate. (Unfortunately, not all communities have physicians listed by specialty.) You can also get a list of rheumatologists in your area from the nearest office of the Arthritis Foundation, Arthritis Care, or the Arthritis Society. An orthopedic surgeon can be of great help in particular instances; do not hesitate to ask your doctor to arrange a referral.

A word of warning: Some people spend a great deal of time and money doctor shopping. They go from doctor to doctor looking for a cure. Unfortunately, doctor shoppers lose out by not having one physician who can get to know them and build an optimal treatment plan over time. The best advice is to find a doctor you like and stick with him or her. Often, with severe arthritis, nearly all of your care should be provided by a rheumatologist.

Communicating With Your Doctor

For a person with arthritis, it is especially important to establish and maintain good communication with the doctor. The relationship you have with your physician must be looked on as a long-term one requiring regular work, much like a business partnership or a marriage.

Your doctor will probably know more intimate details about you than anyone except perhaps your spouse. In turn, you should feel comfortable expressing your fears, asking questions that you may think are "stupid," and negotiating a treatment plan to satisfy you both, without feeling that your doctor is putting you down or is not interested.

There are two things to keep in mind that will help to open, and keep open, the lines of communication with your doctor. How does the doctor feel? Too often we expect our doctor to act as a warmhearted computer—to be a gigantic brain, stuffed with knowledge about the human body, able to analyze the situation and produce a diagnosis, prognosis, and treatment on demand—*and* to be a warm, caring person who makes us feel we are the only person he or she is interested in taking care of.

Actually, most doctors wish they were just that sort of person. But no doctor can be all things to all patients. Doctors are human, too. They get headaches, they get tired, and they get sore feet. They have families who demand their time and attention, and they have to fight bureaucracies as formidable as those the rest of us face.

Most doctors entered the grueling medical training system because they wanted to make sick people well. It is frustrating for them not to be able to cure someone with a chronic condition like arthritis or fibromyalgia. They must take their satisfaction from seeing improvements rather than cures, or even in managing the maintenance of existing conditions and preventing declines. Undoubtedly, you have been frustrated, angry, or depressed from time to time about your condition, but bear in mind that your doctor has probably felt similar emotions about his or her inability to cure you. In this, you are truly partners.

In this partnership between you and your doctor, the biggest threat to a good relationship and good communication is lack of time. If you or your doctor could have a fantasy about the best thing to happen in your relationship, it would probably involve more time for you both: more time to discuss things, more time to explain things, more time to explore options. A doctor is usually on a tight schedule. Doctors try to stay on schedule, but sometimes patients and doctors alike end up feeling rushed, such as when you have to wait in a doctor's office because of an emergency that delays your appointment. When time is short, the result can be rushed messages that are just plain misunderstood—with no time to correct them.

Taking P.A.R.T.
One way you can get the most from your visit with the doctor is to practice what we call P.A.R.T.

| Prepare | Ask | Repeat | Take action |

Prepare
Before visiting or calling your doctor, prepare your agenda. What are the reasons for your visit? What do you expect from your doctor?

Take some time to make a written list of your concerns or questions. Be realistic. If you have thirteen different problems, it isn't likely that your doctor can adequately deal with that many concerns in one visit. Identify your two to four main concerns or problems. Writing them down also helps you remember them. Have you ever thought to yourself, after you walked out of the doctor's office, "Why didn't I ask about . . . ?" or "I forgot to mention . . . . " Making a list beforehand helps ensure that your main concerns get addressed. Also bring a list of all medications you are taking and their dosages. This saves time for other things.

Mention your main concerns right at the beginning of the visit. Don't wait until the end of the appointment to bring up important concerns, because there won't be enough time to deal with them properly. Give your list to the doctor. If the list is long, expect that only two or three items will be addressed on this visit, and let your doctor know which items are the most important to you. Studies show that doctors allow an average of eighteen seconds for the patient to state his or her concerns before interrupting with focused questioning. Preparing your questions in advance will help you use your eighteen seconds well.

Here's an example of bringing up your concerns at the beginning of the visit:

Doctor: What brings you in today?

You: I have a lot of things I want to discuss this visit. (Looking at his or her watch and appointment schedule, the doctor immediately begins to feel anxious.) But I know that we have a limited amount of time. The things that most concern me are my shoulder pain and the side effects from one of the medications I'm taking. (The doctor feels relieved because the concerns are focused and potentially manageable within the appointment time available.)

Try to be as open as you can in sharing your thoughts, feelings, and fears. Your physician is not a mind reader. If you are worried, try to explain why. "I am afraid that I'll become disabled from this," or "My father had similar symptoms and they got worse." The more open you are, the more likely that your doctor can help you.

Give your physician feedback. If you don't like the way you have been treated by the physician or someone else on the health-care team, let your physician know. If you were unable to follow the physician's advice or had problems with a treatment, tell your physician so adjustments can be made. Also, most physicians appreciate compliments and positive feedback, but patients are often hesitant to praise their doctors. So if you are pleased, remember to let your physician know it.

Preparing for a visit involves more than just listing your concerns. You should be prepared to describe your symptoms to the doctor concisely (when they started, how long they last, where they are located, what makes them better or worse, whether you have had similar problems before, whether you have changed your exercise or medications in a way that might contribute to the symptoms, and so on). Only you know the trends and tempo of your arthritis. If you've tried a treatment, you should be prepared to report the effect of the treatment. And if you have previous records or test results that might be relevant to your problems, bring them along. Plan ahead so you can be brief and use your time effectively.

Ask

Another key to effective doctor-patient communication is asking questions. Getting understandable answers and information is one of the cornerstones of self-management. You need to be prepared to ask questions about diagnosis, tests, treatments, and follow-up.

1. **Diagnosis.** Ask your doctor what's wrong, what caused the problem, what is the future outlook (or prognosis), and what can be done to prevent the problem in the future.

2. **Tests.** Ask your doctor if any medical tests are necessary, how they will affect your treatment, how accurate they are, and what is likely to happen if you are not tested. If you decide to have a test, find out how

to prepare for the test, what it will entail, and how to get the results.

3. **Treatments.** Ask about your treatment options, including lifestyle change, medications, and surgery. Inquire about the risks and benefits of treatment and the consequences of not treating.

4. **Follow-up.** Find out if and when you should call or return for a follow-up visit. What symptoms should you watch for and what should you do if they occur?

You may wish to take some notes on important points during the visit or consider bringing along someone else to act as a second listener. Another set of eyes and ears may help you recall later some of the details of the visit or instruction.

Repeat

It is extremely helpful to repeat back briefly to the doctor some of the key points from the visit and discussion. These might include diagnosis, prognosis, next steps, or treatment actions. This is to double-check that you understand the most important information, giving the doctor a chance quickly to correct any misunderstandings and miscommunications. If you don't understand or remember something the physician said, admit that you need to go over it again. Don't be afraid to ask what you may consider a stupid question. You might say, "I'm pretty sure you told me some of this before, but I'm still confused about it." These questions can often indicate an important concern or misunderstanding.

Take Action

When the visit ends, you need to clearly understand what to do next. When appropriate, ask your physician to write down instructions or recommend reading material for more information on a particular subject.

If for some reason you can't or won't follow the doctor's advice, let the doctor know. For example, "I didn't take the aspirin. It gives me stomach problems," or "My insurance doesn't cover that much physical therapy, so I can't afford it," or "I've tried to exercise before, but I can't seem to keep it up." If your doctor knows why you can't or won't follow advice, alternative suggestions can sometimes be made to help you overcome the barrier. If you don't share the barriers to taking actions, it's difficult for your doctor to help.

Asking for a Second Opinion

Many people find it uncomfortable to talk to their doctor about getting a second opinion about their diagnosis or treatment. Especially if patients have a long relationship with their doctor or simply like the doctor, they sometimes worry that asking for another opinion might be interpreted by the doctor as questioning his or her competence. It is a rare doctor whose feelings will be hurt by a sincere request for another opinion. If your condition is medically complicated or difficult, the doctor may have already consulted with another doctor (or more) about your case, at least on an informal basis.

Even if your arthritis is not particularly complicated, asking for a second opinion is a perfectly acceptable, and often expected, request. Doctors prefer a straightforward request. Asking in the form of a nonthreatening "I" message will make this task simple: "I'm still feeling confused and uncomfortable about this treatment. I feel another opinion might help me feel more reassured. Can you suggest someone I could consult?"

In this way, you have expressed your own feelings without suggesting that the doctor is at fault. You have also confirmed your confidence in him or her by asking that he or she suggest the other doctor. (Remember, however, that you are not bound by your doctor's suggestion; you may choose anyone you wish to give you a second opinion.)

Problems

Over the years, we have heard many complaints about doctors and would like to discuss a few of these.

1. "All my doctor does is try one medication after another."

Unfortunately, there is no way your physician can know for sure what medication will work for you. You may need to try a number of medications before you find the right combination.

This trial-and-error method can be expensive. Therefore, when you start a new medication, ask how long it will be until you know whether the drug will be good for you. If you will know in a short time, request a prescription for only a week or two, with refills of the prescription permitted. In this way you can try the medication, and if it doesn't work you won't have a lot of expensive pills to throw away. Sometimes the doctor will have free sample packages available.

Don't be discouraged if you have to try several different medications. Also, don't hesitate to let your doctor know if you have problems with a medication or if it is not working. If you have a problem with a drug and do not have an appointment in the near future, contact your doctor by phone or email.

2. "My doctor never tells me anything about my medications."

Time is often a factor, or maybe you didn't ask. If you want more information about your medications, first ask your physician. If his or her answer is not satisfactory, ask the pharmacist. Pharmacists are an underutilized resource for drug information. Also, this book answers some of the most common questions (see chapters 18, 19, and 20).

3. "There is no cure; there is nothing my doctor can do anyway."

Yes and no. While it is true there is no cure for many types of arthritis and fibromyalgia, there is a great deal that can be done. Diabetes is another disease with no cure. However, insulin and appropriate medical care enable diabetics to live nearly normal lives. No diabetic would think of saying that because there is no cure, physicians can't do anything.

For people with arthritis or fibromyalgia, medical attention can do a number of things. First, just knowing what condition is causing one's problems relieves a lot of worry; this in itself is valuable. Second, physicians may be able to prescribe treatment to make life easier. Third, with many types of arthritis, medical treatment can control the disease or keep it from progressing. Thus, while it is true that doctors often can't cure your condition, they often can help you help yourself to live more comfortably.

4. "My doctor uses language I can't understand."

Unfortunately, doctors are so used to talking "doctor-talk" that they sometimes exclude the rest of us. They don't do this on purpose or even realize they are doing it. The situation is simple. If you don't understand something, ask. Never be afraid to speak up.

5. "My doctor ignores my ideas about self-care."

Now, this is a hard one. Often doctors are not trained in the use of alternative therapies, and, like all of us, they tend to downplay things they don't know about. On the other hand, physicians have a responsibility to let you know when a proposed treatment has little scientific merit or is just plain harmful. At our Arthritis Center in

Stanford, California, we get hundreds of calls a year about all kinds of treatments. We tell people what we know or don't know and try to warn them of possible harm. We, and your doctor, also feel a responsibility to prevent folks from spending large amounts of money on potentially harmful or ineffective treatments.

If your doctor disregards your ideas, then you have an extra responsibility to find out about the treatment. Generally, if the treatment is free or inexpensive and does not have harmful side effects, go ahead and try it if you wish. On the other hand, be very skeptical of expensive treatments (someone is making money off of you). Treatments that promise a cure, or anything with the word *miracle* attached to it, are *never* miracle cures!

6. "My doctor never listens to me."

A good relationship takes two people, people who have similar ideas and are able to communicate. If you feel your doctor is not listening to you, we suggest you discuss it. You can start by saying something like, "Dr. Jones, sometimes I feel I'm not being heard." This takes some nerve, but we can promise that it will open up the communication process.

Another way to get your doctor to listen is to be brief and to the point. You might even practice before going in. Think out exactly what you want to say; this will make it easier.

7. "I don't feel comfortable talking with my doctor."

This is a problem many of us have. We have already discussed many ways you can make communication easier. Here is one more. Whenever you want to have a serious conversation with your doctor, plan to do it while you are dressed. It is hard to feel comfortable in your underwear or an examination gown.

Sometimes the personalities of the physician and the patient just don't fit. If you have tried to open up communication and it hasn't worked, then maybe it is time to find a new doctor. Not every patient can like every doctor and vice versa. Doctors sometimes wish they had the option of changing patients. You do have this option; when necessary, don't be afraid to use it. Good patient-physician relationships are important.

A Note for the Year 2006 and Beyond

In all countries, health systems are changing. Many of these changes are positive. Treatments for arthritis have improved and the future looks even brighter. On the other hand, getting health care is often more complex. Many of us see more than one physician. In the past, we assumed that somehow, when we were referred from one physician to another, all our information went with us. As the health-care system gets more and more complex, this is seldom true. In fact, it is more important than ever that we are well informed about our care and are able to pass this information on to new health professionals. Keep a record of your medications, recent laboratory results, and other information about your health. Be ready to give these to each new health professional. One way to be sure information gets to a new doctor is to carry it. Also, if you have had laboratory tests and not received the results, ask for them. Never assume that no news is good news. By being a proactive self-manager, you can be assured that you will not be lost in the system and that each of your health-care providers will have current information. Be prepared to do your part to get the best care possible.

A Doctor's Addendum

I have never seen a person with arthritis or fibromyalgia I couldn't help. There are some individuals, however, whom I have not helped. In every such case, the communication broke down. Sometimes I am short of time or short of temper. Sometimes the person doesn't listen or doesn't hear or doesn't understand. Often, a preconceived opinion is the problem: "Aspirin won't work"; "My neighbor couldn't tolerate that drug"; "I hardly eat a thing"; "She seems too old to exercise"; "I don't think he would understand." Or a person never filled a prescription, stopped an exercise program after two days, decreased medication ("It was too expensive"), and never mentioned the problem. A solid half of the blame lies with the doctor. Sometimes we do not listen, or we have our own preconceived ideas. No matter how hard we try we don't always get it right. But the other half of the blame lies with the patient. Tell it true and straight, and we can help. This is a partnership. We don't always have to agree to get good results. But the give-and-take of direct communication is essential.

Chapter 18

The Drug Scene: Medicines to Reduce Pain and Inflammation

Recently there has been an unprecedented explosion of new and different treatments for arthritis. Some are safer than previously available alternatives, some use entirely new approaches to arthritis relief, and some give better results for some—but not all—patients. However, some don't work, and others have been found to be harmful. The period beginning in 1998 has brought the most exciting wave of new arthritis treatments ever seen. This is generally good news for patients, but both doctors and patients need to learn about the new drugs and how to use them wisely.

Knowing all about your drugs is important, but it is not easy. Drugs have complex effects on your body, some good and some bad, and a full explanation from your doctor always takes lots of time. Unfortunately that time is not always available in the modern doctor visit, which is all too brief. The interview with your doctor is an intensive experience, and detailed discussion of prescribed treatment is often neglected. Little time is spent on the important subject of how to use your medications correctly. In chapters 18, 19, and 20, the discussions you've been having with your physician are repeated. Read the ones you need. Reread those you've forgotten.

The internet makes it both easier and harder to learn about medicines. Much of the information is inaccurate or not appropriate for your problem. "Direct to Consumer" drug advertising can be very misleading and full of "spin."

There are four major types of arthritis medications. First, there are drugs that both moderate inflammation and reduce pain, nonsteroidal anti-inflammatory drugs (NSAIDs). Second, there are corticosteroid hormone anti-inflammatory medications. Third, there are strongly anti-inflammatory disease-modifying antirheumatic drugs (DMARDs), which improve the overall course of an inflammatory arthritis such as rheumatoid arthritis. And fourth, there are drugs that are analgesic only, directed at relieving pain. We discuss the first two types in this chapter, and the third and fourth in Chapter 19 and Chapter 20, respectively.

Common Anti-inflammatory Medications (NSAIDs)

Inflammation

The pain, swelling, and joint destruction caused by many kinds of arthritis are a result of inflammation around the joint. Many important arthritis medicines are intended to reduce inflammation. Yet inflammation is part of the body's normal healing process. When injured, the body increases blood flow to the injured area and sends inflammatory cells to repair the wounded tissue and to kill bacterial invaders. The inflammation causes the area to be warm, red, tender, and often swollen. Inflammation is a normal process and can often be helpful rather than harmful.

In osteoarthritis there is little inflammation, or the inflammation may be necessary for the healing process. But in rheumatoid arthritis, psoriatic arthritis, ankylosing spondylitis, and other inflammatory forms of arthritis, the inflammation itself causes damage; thus, suppression of the inflammation can be helpful in treatment. You don't always want the minor NSAIDs just because you have arthritis: in osteoarthritis, often no; in rheumatoid arthritis, you want stronger anti-inflammatories, usually DMARDs.

Nonsteroidal Anti-inflammatory Drugs (NSAIDs) and Aspirin

The first NSAID was aspirin, introduced in 1898. Chewing on willow bark, which contains salicylate, to relieve pain had been practiced for several hundred years before that. The newer NSAIDs began to arrive in the mid-1960s when Indocin, Motrin, Naprosyn, Tolectin, and Nalfon became available. Many, many NSAIDs have been introduced since. Some work better than others for particular patients. Some have more side effects than others. In low doses these drugs are analgesic; that is, they relieve pain. In higher doses they also reduce inflammation.

These drugs have important roles beyond the treatment of arthritis. Low-dose aspirin is effective in preventing heart attacks. It appears that some NSAIDs, including aspirin, are useful in preventing colon cancer, and some may even slow the development of Alzheimer's disease.

NSAIDs work by blocking the enzyme cyclooxygenase (COX), which stimulates inflammation. The major side effects of these drugs come from the same blocking of the COX enzyme. The drugs deplete a protective chemical, prostaglandin, in the wall of the stomach and other parts of the gastrointestinal (GI) tract. As a result, ulcers can form, and these can cause serious bleeding from the stomach as well as other complications. Because NSAIDs are so widely used, over 50,000 hospitalizations in the United States and over 5,000 deaths each year are caused by the gastrointestinal side effects of these drugs. The people most likely to get these side effects are older, more disabled, taking higher doses of the drugs, taking the drugs for longer periods, and taking prednisone at the same time. They also have had previous side effects with drugs of this class.

Since recognition of the problem of "NSAID gastropathy" some ten years ago, largely as a result of research by our group, there has been a search for less toxic NSAIDs and for treatments that can block side effects. This search has been largely successful. First, misoprostil (Cytotec) was introduced. Misoprostil itself is a prostaglandin and replaces the lost prostaglandin in the stomach wall, preventing many problems. Unfortunately, it often causes diarrhea. After misoprostil, less toxic NSAIDs were discovered. These were less acidic or were somewhat safer for other reasons. Rheumatologists now often use lower NSAID doses or use Tylenol instead.

The most recent approach toward safer NSAIDs has come from a new scientific discovery. The enzyme COX has been found to be two enzymes, now called COX-1 and COX-2. The side effects come almost entirely from blockage of the COX-1 enzyme, and the desired antiinflammatory effects from blockage of COX-2. New drugs, called selective COX-2 inhibitors, preserve most of the desired effects while eliminating most of the undesired ones. Actually the new drugs would be better termed "COX-1 sparing" drugs, since these drugs are *not* more powerful anti-inflammatory agents than older drugs. Their effectiveness is about the same. The advantage of the newer drugs is greater safety for the stomach. Tragically, they have other, perhaps more severe, side effects.

NSAIDs and Side Effects

All NSAIDs used to be thought equal in toxicity. Then research, first by our research group and later by others, proved that there were big differences in the frequency of side effects with different NSAIDs. The table on pages

262–263 lists NSAIDs, grouped by the frequency of serious gastrointestinal (GI) side effects. The individual drugs are discussed in more detail later in this chapter. Misoprostil, which can be combined with any of the NSAIDs, is discussed under Arthrotec. The groupings in the table are consistent with recent research. On average, the most toxic NSAIDs will be three or more times as toxic as the least toxic. Costs are estimated from our data, from the manufacturer's data in some cases, and from the formulary listings of a major national health plan. Within groupings, the drugs are listed in alphabetical order. The least toxic drugs are increasing in use, the most toxic are decreasing.

If you are taking one of the more toxic NSAIDs, or even one of the moderately toxic ones, you might want to discuss with your doctor whether a less toxic NSAID might work just as well. Remember, all drugs can cause side effects, and the safety of any drug is only relative compared with others. Different people respond better or worse to different drugs.

Here are some hints about NSAID side effects. Lower doses of these drugs are always less toxic than higher doses. If you have a serious medical problem such as heart failure, liver disease, or kidney disease, the drugs are likely to be more toxic, and even lower doses may be needed. Generic forms of these drugs are similar in both effectiveness and toxicity to brand-name drugs; they are much less expensive, as can be seen in the table. The more recently introduced drugs are more expensive than the earlier ones, and generic drugs usually are the least expensive. The claim "as safe as aspirin" is misleading; all of these drugs—including aspirin—need to be used carefully and with respect. When two or more drugs are taken, there can be drug interactions that cause other side effects, as with additional toxicity when prednisone is taken at the same time and interferes with blood-thinning medicines such as Coumadin. If you are taking

NSAID Toxicity for
Serious Gastrointestinal (GI) Problems

Nonsteroidal Anti-inflammatory Drug (NSAID)	Estimated Cost (Branded/Generic)
LEAST TOXIC NSAIDS	
Arthrotec (diclofenac and misoprostil)	$$$/–
ASA (aspirin) less than 2600 mg/day*	$/$
Celebrex (celecoxib)	$$$/–
Lodine (etodolac)	$$/–
Mobic (meloxicam)	$$/–
Motrin (ibuprofen)*	$$/$
Relafen (nabumetone)	$$/–
Salsalate (salicylate)*	$$/$$
Trilisate (trisalicylate)*	$$/$$
MODERATELY TOXIC NSAIDS	
Clinoril (sulindac)	$$/$$
Daypro (oxaprozin)	$$/–
Dolobid (diflunisal)	$$/$
Naprosyn (naproxen)*	$$/$

other medicines, you should ask your doctor if any drug interactions with NSAIDs are likely.

What follows in the remainder of this chapter are general recommendations. If your doctor's advice differs, then listen to your doctor. He or she is most familiar with your specific needs. The cautions listed are those known at the time of this writing and are subject to

**NSAID Toxicity for
Serious Gastrointestinal (GI) Problems** *(continued)*

Nonsteroidal Anti-inflammatory Drug (NSAID)	Estimated Cost (Branded/Generic)
MODERATELY TOXIC NSAIDS *(continued)*	
Orudis (ketoprofen)*	$$/$
Voltaren (diclofenac)	$$$/$$
MOST TOXIC NSAIDS	
Ansaid (flurbiprofen)	$$/–
Feldene (piroxicam)	$$/$
Indocin (indomethacin)	$/$
Meclomen (meclofenamate)	$$/$$
Tolectin (tolmetin)	$$/$$

$$$	most expensive
$$	moderately expensive
$	least expensive
*	available over the counter
–	not available in generic product

NOTE: Tylenol (acetaminophen), which is analgesic only, would be among the least toxic and least expensive.

changes that your doctor may know about. But if you receive advice that doesn't make sense according to the principles outlined in this section, don't hesitate to ask questions or get another opinion.

Finally, these drugs are big business and the marketing "spin" has been very misleading. There is a strong tendency to overhype new and expensive drugs. The newer drugs, the coxibs, have been touted as much safer than older drugs, but they are no safer than many older drugs (and they may cause heart attacks). They are frequently termed "COX-2's" but all NSAIDs (old and new) inhibit COX-2 about equally.

Aspirin and Other Salicylates

Acetylsalicylic acid (aspirin)
Purpose: To relieve pain; to reduce inflammation. Oldest, cheapest, and still good.

Indications: Pain relief for osteoarthritis, rheumatoid arthritis, and local conditions such as bursitis. Anti-inflammatory agent for rheumatoid arthritis if taken in high doses. In low doses (81 mg/day) prevents heart attacks. May prevent colon cancer.

Dosage: For pain, two 5-grain tablets (5 grains equals 325 mg) every four hours as needed. For anti-inflammatory action, three to four tablets, four to six times daily (with medical supervision if these doses are continued for longer than one week). The time to maximum effect is thirty minutes to one hour for pain and one to three weeks for the anti-inflammatory action.

Side effects: Common effects include nausea, vomiting, ringing in the ears, and decreased hearing. Each of these is reversible within a few hours if the drug dosage is decreased. Allergic reactions are rare but include development of nasal polyps and wheezing. With an overdose of aspirin there is very rapid and heavy breathing, and there can even be unconsciousness and coma. Be sure to keep aspirin (and all medications) out of the reach of children.

Aspirin has some predictable effects that occur in just about everyone. Blood loss through the bowel occurs in almost all persons who take aspirin, because the blood clotting function is decreased, the stomach is irritated, and aspirin acts as a blood-thinning agent. Since serious liver damage does not occur, routine blood tests to check for this complication usually are not required. Hospitalization for gastrointestinal hemorrhage occurs in about 1% of people taking full doses for one year.

Aspirin is not recommended for children with influenza, chicken pox, or high fevers because of the possibility of a rare liver and brain complication called Reye syndrome.

Special hints: Aspirin remains an important drug for treatment of arthritis. If you note ringing in the ears or a decrease in your hearing, then decrease the dose of aspirin. Your dose is just a little bit too high for the best result. Some people develop nasal polyps or wheezing with salicylates; if you are one of those people, these drugs are not for you.

If you notice nausea, an upset stomach, or vomiting, there are a variety of things you can do. First, try spreading out the dose with more frequent use of smaller numbers of pills. Perhaps instead of taking four tablets four times a day, you might take three tablets five or six times a day. Second, try taking the aspirin after meals or after an antacid, which will coat the stomach and provide some protection. Third, you can change brands and see if the nausea is related to the particular brand of aspirin you are using. Fourth, you can try coated aspirin (Ecotrin).

If you are taking high doses or are at risk for GI bleeding, talk with your doctor about using a proton pump inhibitor (PPI) to protect the stomach. This advice holds for all NSAIDs.

Keep track of your aspirin intake and always tell your doctor exactly how much you are taking. Aspirin is so familiar that sometimes we forget we are taking a drug. Be as careful with aspirin as you would be with any other drug. In particular you may want to ask your doctor about interactions with the newer anti-inflammatory agents, with probenecid, or with blood-thinning drugs. Pay special attention to your stomach. So many drugs cause irritation to the stomach lining that you run the risk of adding insult to injury. Two drugs that irritate the stomach lining may be more than twice as dangerous as one. Again, the fewer medications taken at one time the better. Every time you talk to a doctor, be sure to describe all the drugs you are taking, not just your arthritis drugs. It is wise to keep a list of all the drugs you take and have it ready to show any doctor you visit, including your dentist.

Disalcid (salsalate)
500 mg round, aqua, scored, film-coated tablet
500 mg aqua and white capsule
750 mg capsule-shaped, aqua, scored, film-coated tablet

Ecotrin
325 mg, 500 mg tablet or caplet
See acetylsalicylic acid (aspirin)

Trilisate (choline magnesium trisalicylate)
500 mg capsule-shaped, pale pink, scored tablet
750 mg capsule-shaped, white, scored, film-coated tablet
1,000 mg capsule-shaped, red, scored, film-coated tablet

Purpose: These aspirin-like drugs are to relieve pain; to reduce inflammation.

Indications: For mild pain relief of cartilage degeneration and local conditions. Also anti-inflammatory agents.

Dosage: For pain, one or two 500 mg tablets every twelve hours. For anti-inflammatory activity, 1,000 to 1,500 mg every twelve hours. Occasionally higher doses may be needed. The maximum effect is reached in two hours for pain effects; one to three weeks are required for anti-inflammatory action to take full effect. In higher doses and for courses of more than two weeks, check with your doctor.

Side effects: Common effects include nausea, vomiting, ringing in the ears, and decreased hearing. Each of these is reversible within a few hours if the drug dosage is decreased. Allergic reactions are rare but may include development of nasal polyps and wheezing. With an overdose of salicylate there can be very heavy and rapid breathing, which can lead to unconsciousness and coma.

Non-Aspirin NSAIDs

There is a huge market for NSAIDs. Nearly every major drug company has tried to invent one and has promoted heavily whatever has been developed. Most recently, new drugs have been promoted as "coxibs," "selective Cox-two inhibitors," or even "Cox-2's." But, they are just NSAIDs, no more powerful, a little easier on the stomach, but some have been found to increase risk for heart attacks.

The same "possible heart attack risk" problem exists for possible future "coxibs" such as lumiricoxib and etoricoxib as with the current drug celecoxib. Vioxx, an earlier coxib (rofecoxib), and valdecoxib (Bextra) were removed from the market for this problem. We personally will not use any of these "coxibs" except in very low cardiac risk patients (age under 50, no major disease, short-term use) until their safety is confirmed by good, large, long-term studies.

Commonly Used NSAIDs
Arthrotec, Celebrex, Clinoril, Daypro, Feldene, Indocin, Lodine, Mobic, Motrin, Naprosyn, Orudis, Relafen, Voltaren

Available evidence indicates that different drugs work best for different individuals. These drugs come from several different chemical families and are not interchangeable. You may have to try several to find the best. The most frequently used medications in this category are discussed below in alphabetical order, according to brand name. The generic name is given in parentheses.

Advil (ibuprofen)
See Motrin and Ibuprofen. Sold over the counter.

Aleve (naproxen)
See Naprosyn and Naproxen. Sold over the counter.

Arthrotec (diclofenac plus misoprostil)
Tablets with 50 or 75 mg diclofenac and 200 micrograms misoprostil

Purpose: To reduce inflammation; to reduce pain; to reduce gastrointestinal side effects.

Indications: For anti-inflammatory action and pain relief.

Dosage: 50 mg/200 twice daily or three times daily; 75 mg/200 twice daily.

Side effects: Gastrointestinal side effects occur, with the most common being irritation of the stomach lining, nausea, indigestion, and heartburn. Additionally, diarrhea is quite common. Hospitalization for gastrointestinal bleeding occurs in about 0.5% of those taking full doses for one year. Further side effects are discussed under Voltaren.

This is a combination drug, in which misoprostil is included to preserve prostaglandin in the stomach lining and to decrease the chance of serious side effects. It decreases serious side effects from the diclofenac by about half. This is sufficient to make it a safer drug, but probably still not the safest. Unfortunately, the addition of misoprostil also increases the toxicity for diarrhea, and many individuals have diarrhea resulting from the drug. As a result, the relatively minor symptoms such as nausea and diarrhea are not reduced over other drugs, although the serious side effects are.

Special hints: For stomach upset, take the pills after meals and skip a dose or two if necessary. Diarrhea may last only for a short time and may be mild, or it may necessitate reduction in dose or even switching to another drug. Check with your doctor if the distress continues. Maximum therapeutic effect is achieved after one to two weeks of treatment and you should be able to see a major effect in the first week if Arthrotec is going to be a really good drug for you. Drugs likely to be of equal or lesser toxicity for the GI tract include low-dose aspirin, low-dose ibuprofen, Tylenol, Disalcid, Trilisate, Lodine, Relafen, and the COX-1-sparing drugs.

Bextra (valdecoxib)
No longer available because it appeared to cause heart attacks in a few people and was recalled.

Celebrex (celecoxib)
100 mg tablet

Purpose: To reduce inflammation; to reduce pain; to reduce gastrointestinal side effects.

Indications: For anti-inflammatory action and pain relief.

Dosage: For osteoarthritis, 200 mg daily or 100 mg twice daily; for rheumatoid arthritis, 100–200 mg twice daily.

Side effects: Minor gastrointestinal side effects are quite common and include nausea, indigestion, heartburn, and diarrhea. Other side effects seen with other NSAIDs are also seen on occasion. This is a COX-1-sparing (selective COX-2 inhibitor) drug. It has been designed to reduce serious gastrointestinal problems. Some studies have suggested a slight increase in heart attacks; others have not.

Special hints: This drug has been described in the lay press as a "super aspirin." However, it is *not* more powerful than previously available drugs. It should be safer. It is a new drug, and some side effects may not yet have been discovered. It may be more expensive than alternatives. It is probably not GI safer than Disalcid, Tylenol, Mobic, or several other drugs. We suggest not using doses above 200 mg/day except in young healthy people.

For stomach upset, take the pills after meals and skip a dose or two if necessary. Antacids may be used for gastrointestinal problems and may help. Check with your doctor if the distress continues. You should be able to see a major effect in the first week or so if Celebrex is going to be a really good drug for you.

Clinoril (sulindac)
150 mg, 200 mg hexagon-shaped, bright yellow tablet

Purpose: To reduce inflammation; to reduce pain.

Indications: For anti-inflammatory action and pain relief.

Dosage: One 150 mg tablet twice a day. This drug also comes in a 200 mg tablet and dosage may be increased to 200 mg twice a day if needed. Maximum recommended dose is 400 mg a day.

Side effects: Gastrointestinal side effects, with irritation of the stomach lining, are the most common, and include nausea, indigestion, and heartburn. Stomach pain has been reported in 10% of subjects, and nausea, diarrhea, constipation, headache, and rash in 3 to 9%. Ringing in the ears, fluid retention, itching, and nervousness have been reported. Allergic reactions are rare. The manufacturer does not recommend the use of aspirin in combination with this drug since aspirin apparently decreases absorption from the intestine. Hospitalization for gastrointestinal bleeding occurs in about 1% of those taking full doses for one year.

Special hints: Sulindac has no particular advantages over the other anti-inflammatory agents described in this section, except that it may cause the minor kidney side effects less frequently and therefore is sometimes used for people with heart or kidney problems. It is of moderate toxicity.

For stomach upset, take the pills after meals; skip a dose or two if necessary. Check with your doctor if the distress continues. Maximum therapeutic effect is achieved after about three weeks of treatment, but you should be able to see a major effect in the first week if sulindac is going to be a really good drug for you.

Daypro (oxaprozin)
600 mg caplet

Purpose: To reduce inflammation; to reduce pain.

Indications: For anti-inflammatory action and pain relief in osteoarthritis and rheumatoid arthritis.

Dosage: The usual daily dose in rheumatoid arthritis or severe osteoarthritis is 1,200 mg (two 600 mg caplets) taken once daily. For patients of lower body weight or with milder disease, an initial dosage of one 600 mg caplet per day might be appropriate.

Side effects: Daypro can cause serious side effects, including stomach ulcers and intestinal bleeding. Most common side effects are dyspepsia and abdominal pain. As with other NSAIDs, serious side effects, such as gastrointestinal bleeding, may result in hospitalization or even fatal outcomes.

Special hints: Daypro's overall toxicity is probably about average. It has no particular advantages over other NSAIDs, although some people respond well to it. It should not be taken by pregnant or nursing women. Its principal feature is that it needs to be taken only once a day, since it has a long half-life. This is a convenience feature but it does suggest caution in dosage, particularly if the patient is older or has other disease problems, since the drug might accumulate in the body. The maximum daily dose is 1,800 mg, but this is seldom used.

Feldene (piroxicam)
10 mg dark red and blue capsule, 20 mg dark red capsule

Purpose: To reduce inflammation; to reduce pain.

Indications: For anti-inflammatory activity and mild pain in rheumatoid arthritis, local conditions, and sometimes osteoarthritis.

Dosage: One 10 or 20 mg tablet once daily. Do not exceed this dosage. This is a long-acting drug, and it needs to be taken only once daily. We suggest using only the 10 mg tablet.

Side effects: The drug has been consistently recognized as one of the more toxic NSAIDs. Gastrointestinal symptoms that involve irritation of the stomach lining occur, including nausea, indigestion, and heartburn. Allergic reactions, including skin rashes and asthma, are rare. Peptic ulceration can occur, and hospitalization for gastrointestinal bleeding is seen in about 2% of those who take full doses for one year. Because Feldene is so long lasting, it may be unusually toxic for elderly people or for people with liver and kidney problems.

Special hints: Some seven to twelve days are required before the benefits of Feldene are apparent, and full benefits may not be clear for six weeks or more. Aspirin, except in low dose, should be avoided. Dosage recommendations and indications for use in children have not been established. Some patients with rheumatoid arthritis or osteoarthritis prefer Feldene, particularly because of the convenience of the once-a-day dosage. Feldene is declining in use.

Indocin (indomethacin)
25 mg, 50 mg blue and white capsule
75 mg blue and white, sustained-release capsule
50 mg blue suppository

Purpose: To reduce inflammation; to reduce pain.

Indications: For reduction of inflammation and for pain relief.

Dosage: One 25 mg capsule three to four times daily. For some patients, doses totaling as high as 150 mg (six capsules) may be required each day. Indocin is also available in 50 mg capsules. The 75 mg sustained-release form needs to be taken only twice daily (and no more).

Side effects: Irritation of the stomach lining, including nausea, indigestion, and heartburn, occurs in a number of people. Allergic reactions (including skin rash and asthma) are rare. A substantial problem, not present with other drugs of this class, is headache and a bit of a goofy feeling. Hospitalization for gastrointestinal bleeding is seen in about 2% of those on full doses for one year. Indocin is one of the more toxic NSAIDs.

Special hints: Many doctors find Indocin to be rather weak for treatment of rheumatoid arthritis. Maximum effect may take three weeks or so, but you should be able to tell within one week if it is going to be a major help.

Some studies suggest that Indocin actually *increases* the rate of cartilage destruction in osteoarthritis of the hip. Usually it should not be the first NSAID tried.

Indocin, despite its potential toxicity, is often very effective in ankylosing spondylitis, Reiter's syndrome, and psoriatic arthritis. If you take it after meals you will have less stomach irritation, but some people do not absorb the drug very well. So for maximum effect, you need to take it on an empty stomach, and for maximum comfort, take it on a full stomach. Trial and error may be necessary to establish the best regimen for you. When some individuals take aspirin with Indocin, the Indocin is not absorbed from the intestine. Usually you will not want to take these two drugs together since you will get more irritation of the stomach lining but no more therapeutic effect. If this drug makes you feel mentally or emotionally fuzzy for more than the first few weeks, we think that is a good reason to discuss a change in medication with your doctor.

Lodine (etodolac)
200 mg capsule, light gray with one red band or dark gray with two narrow red bands
300 mg capsule, light gray with two narrow red bands

Purpose: To reduce inflammation; to reduce pain.

Indications: For anti-inflammatory action and pain relief.

Dosage: For osteoarthritis, initially 800 to 1,200 mg per day in several doses. Do not exceed 1,200 mg per day. Lodine is not currently recommended for rheumatoid arthritis.

Side effects: This drug is generally well tolerated, although, as with all of the nonsteroidal agents, it can result in bleeding from the stomach and other gastrointestinal problems. Some studies suggest there are fewer ulcers with this drug than with some other NSAIDs; thus, it is relatively safe.

Special hints: Lodine is one of the newer nonsteroidal drugs. More studies are needed to determine its usefulness when compared with other nonsteroidal anti-inflammatory drugs. Lodine has been found less useful in treating rheumatoid arthritis than other drugs of this class. It does have some advantages with regard to gastrointestinal toxicity, and serious side effects are relatively rare.

Mobic (meloxicam)
7.5 mg tablet

Purpose: To reduce inflammation; to reduce pain; to reduce serious gastrointestinal side effects.

Indications: For anti-inflammatory action and pain relief.

Dosage: One or two 7.5 mg tablets daily.

Side effects: This is a preferential COX-1-sparing drug. As such, it is likely to have fewer serious gastrointestinal reactions than other drugs. In high doses (22.5 to 30 mg daily—not recommended), it appears to be as toxic as the typical NSAID. At recommended doses it appears to be one of the safest agents and does not appear to increase heart attack risk.

Relatively minor gastrointestinal side effects such as nausea, indigestion, and heartburn are reasonably common. Allergic reactions are rare and the drug is generally among the best tolerated.

Special hints: Mobic's principal advantage is that of relative safety, although how this safety compares with that of the other less toxic NSAIDs is not established. Considerable international experience suggests that it is moderately effective and comparatively well tolerated. It is a long-acting drug and needs to be taken only once daily. With side effects, reduce the dose or skip a few days. If symptoms persist, check with your doctor. Aspirin, except in very low doses, should not be taken with Mobic. Maximum effect is achieved after about two weeks of treatment.

Motrin (ibuprofen)
300 mg round, white tablet
400 mg round, red-orange tablet
600 mg oval, peach tablet
800 mg capsule-shaped, apricot tablet

Motrin, Advil, and Rufen are the same drug, ibuprofen, produced by different companies. The over-the-counter brands contain smaller doses of ibuprofen (200 mg) and are available without a prescription (see next section).

Purpose: To reduce inflammation; to reduce pain.

Indications: For anti-inflammatory action and pain relief.

Dosage: One or two 400 mg tablets three times daily. Maximum daily recommended dosage is 2,400 mg, or six tablets.

Side effects: Motrin has fewer serious side effects than the other "older" NSAIDs. Gastrointestinal side effects, with irritation of the stomach lining, are the most common, and include nausea, indigestion, and heartburn. Allergic reactions are rare and the drug is generally well tolerated. A very few individuals have been observed with aseptic meningitis, apparently related to this drug. Here the person experiences a headache, fever, and stiff neck, and examination of the spinal fluid shows an increase in spinal fluid protein and white blood cells. The syndrome goes away when the drug is stopped but can come back if the drug is given again. Occasionally individuals may retain fluid with this medication. Hospitalization for gastrointestinal bleeding is needed in about 0.5% of those who take full doses of 2,400 mg per day or more for one year.

Special hints: Motrin is not consistently useful for the treatment of rheumatoid arthritis. Overall, many doctors feel that it is one of the weaker therapeutic agents in this group. If you are not getting enough relief, you may wish to discuss a change in medication with your doctor. Avoidance of Motrin while taking aspirin is strongly advised. Motrin interferes with the actions of aspirin, including cardioprotection. We do not recommend its use in people taking aspirin to protect against heart attacks except for very short periods.

Maximum effect is achieved after about three weeks of treatment, but if it is going to be a really good drug for you, you should be able to see a major effect in the first week.

Ibuprofen Sold Over the Counter

The Food and Drug Administration has approved the sale of ibuprofen without a prescription in a smaller, 200 mg tablet size. This historic ruling added a third over-the-counter analgesic to aspirin and acetaminophen, and now naproxen (Aleve) and ketoprofen (Orudis) are also available over the counter. Advil, Nuprin, and Motrin are the trade names for over-the-counter ibuprofen, and they are heavily advertised and heavily used. Ibuprofen is now also present in many different over-the-counter medications, including Midol. Remember, NSAIDs should be taken with caution whether prescription or nonprescription. Many serious gastrointestinal problems are seen even in people taking self-prescribed drugs.

What does this availability over the counter mean for the patient with arthritis? Relatively little. Many arthritis patients need at least 2,400 mg of ibuprofen per day, and twelve Advil tablets a day rather than four to six prescription Motrin is a bit of a nuisance. And it is hard to save money since the cost per milligram is about the same by prescription as over the counter. If you need anti-inflammatory doses of ibuprofen, you should be seeing your doctor every so often anyway, so do not use the availability of the product over the counter as an excuse to stay away from the doctor. Also, many health insurance plans will not pay for medication unless it is purchased by prescription. Our recommendation remains that ibuprofen for arthritis be used on a prescription basis unless just an occasional tablet is required for pain. Similar advice holds for naproxen or ketoprofen. Remember, do not use ibuprofen except briefly if you are taking aspirin to protect your heart; ibuprofen can block this heart protection.

Naprosyn (naproxen)

250 mg round, light yellow tablet
375 mg capsule-shaped, peach tablet
500 mg capsule-shaped, light yellow tablet

Purpose: To reduce inflammation; to reduce pain.

Indications: For anti-inflammatory action and pain relief.

Dosage: One tablet two or three times a day. Maximum recommended dosage is 1,000 mg a day.

Side effects: Gastrointestinal side effects, with irritation of the stomach lining, are the most common, and include nausea, indigestion, and heartburn. Skin rash and other allergic problems are very rare. Fluid retention has been reported in a few individuals. Hospitalization for gastrointestinal bleeding is required in approximately 1% of patients taking full doses for one year, making it about average in toxicity.

Special hints: Naprosyn has an advantage over some drugs in this class by having a longer half-life. Each tablet lasts eight to twelve hours. Thus, you do not have to take as many tablets as with the other medicines in this group. Naprosyn is one of the most popular of the drugs of this class. Generic naproxen is now available, since the original naproxen patent has expired, and is much less expensive. Naproxen is believed by many rheumatologists to be more effective than most other NSAIDs.

In general, if you are taking Naprosyn you should avoid aspirin, since it interferes with Naprosyn in some individuals. An exception: Small doses of aspirin (e.g., 81 mg per day) used to thin the blood and prevent heart attacks may be used with Naprosyn. If you notice fluid retention, reduce your salt and sodium intake and discuss a change in medication with your doctor. If you have stomach irritation, try taking the tablets on a full stomach or after antacids. Although absorption may be slightly decreased, you may be more comfortable overall.

Naproxen Sold Over the Counter

In 1993 the Food and Drug Administration (FDA) approved naproxen for nonprescription use in a smaller (200 mg) tablet size, adding a fourth over-the-counter pain reliever to the previously available acetaminophen, aspirin, and ibuprofen. Its longer half-life means that it only needs to be taken every eight to twelve hours. You should not take more than three tablets in twenty-four hours (people over age 65 should not exceed two tablets) except on your doctor's recommendation. As with over-the-counter ibuprofen, we believe that most arthritis patients should be using prescription naproxen under a doctor's supervision.

Nuprin (ibuprofen)
200 mg yellow tablet or caplet
See Motrin and Ibuprofen. Sold over the counter.

Orudis, Oruvail (ketoprofen)
25 mg dark green and red capsule
50 mg dark green and light green capsule
75 mg dark green and white capsule

Purpose: To reduce inflammation; to reduce pain.

Indications: For anti-inflammatory action and pain relief.

Dosage: Orudis comes in 25 mg, 50 mg, and 75 mg capsules. Recommended daily dose is 150 to 300 mg divided into three or four doses. Oruvail is a more recent variant of Orudis, with a longer half-life.

Side effects: As with other drugs of this group, the most frequent side effects are gastrointestinal. Irritation of the stomach lining can cause nausea, heartburn, and indigestion. Occasionally individuals note fluid retention. Allergic reactions such as rash or asthma are very rare. Hospitalization for gastrointestinal bleeding occurs in over 1% of those taking full doses for one year, making it a bit worse than average in the frequency of serious toxicity.

Special hints: Chemically, Orudis is related to ibuprofen and naproxen. If you experience irritation of the stomach, decrease the dose or spread the tablets out throughout the day. Absorption will be slightly deceased if you take the drugs after meals or antacids, but greater comfort may result. Ketoprofen is useful in rheumatoid arthritis. It has found use in degenerative arthritis of the hip and for treatment of local conditions. Like other drugs of this group, ketoprofen will be the preferred drug by certain individuals. Orudis is now available over the counter. Since it appears to be more toxic than ibuprofen or naproxen, it should probably not be used as an OTC drug of first choice, and should be taken regularly only under a doctor's supervision.

Relafen (nabumetone)
500 mg oval, film-coated tablet
750 mg oval, film-coated tablet

Purpose: To reduce inflammation; to reduce pain.

Indications: For anti-inflammatory action and pain relief in patients with osteoarthritis and rheumatoid arthritis.

Dosage: Therapy is usually initiated at a dose of 1,000 mg daily, then adjusted, if needed, on the basis of clinical response.

Side effects: This is a relatively new drug, and it has been developed in part to minimize toxic effects on the stomach lining. It appears to be among the least toxic NSAIDs, with less than 0.5% serious gastrointestinal events each year. On the other hand, reductions in the frequency of major ulcers and of bleeding from the stomach have not yet been proved beyond doubt. Diarrhea is said to occur in 14% of people with this drug, heartburn in 13%, and abdominal pain in 12%. These figures are not very different from those of other NSAIDs.

Special hints: Do not exceed 2,000 mg per day. The lowest effective dose should be used if you are going to be taking this drug for a while. Many rheumatologists believe this to be a relatively weak NSAID, but safe. It does not appear to increase heart attack risk.

Vioxx (rofecoxib)
Removed from market because of increased numbers of heart attacks in patients taking this drug.

Voltaren, Cataflam (diclofenac)
25 mg round, yellow, film-coated tablet
50 mg round, light brown, film-coated tablet
75 mg round, white, film-coated tablet

Purpose: To reduce inflammation; to reduce pain.

Indications: For anti-inflammatory action and pain relief.

Dosage: Usually one tablet (25 mg, 50 mg, or 75 mg) two or three times a day. The maximum recommended dosage is 200 mg per day.

Side effects: The most frequent side effects are gastrointestinal. As with other drugs of this group, irritation of the stomach lining can cause nausea, heartburn, and indigestion. Occasionally individuals may note fluid retention. Allergic reactions such as rash or asthma are very rare. Hospitalization for gastrointestinal bleeding probably occurs in about 1% of those taking full doses for one year, making it about average in risk for serious toxicity.

Special hints: Voltaren is the most frequently used non-steroidal medication worldwide. The FDA was slow to review it, in part because of fear it would lead to more frequent liver problems. This does not appear to be a major problem, but periodic blood tests for liver toxicity are recommended by some.

Voltaren comes with an "enteric coating" designed to improve stomach tolerance; this is probably not effective. In case of irritation of the stomach, decrease the dose or spread the tablets out throughout the day. Absorption will be slightly decreased if you take the drug after meals or after antacids, but greater comfort may result.

Voltaren is useful in rheumatoid arthritis, degenerative arthritis, and treatment of local conditions. Certain individuals will prefer Voltaren to other drugs of this group. Cataflam is a derivative drug; its uses are in short-term pain relief and not arthritis treatment.

Less Frequently Used NSAIDs
Ansaid, Dolobid, Meclomen, Tolectin, Toradol

A number of NSAIDs have little advantage over alternatives and have gradually fallen into relative disuse. They may, however, have advantages for individual patients, so follow your doctor's advice. They are not discussed in detail here.

Ansaid (flurbiprofen) is an average NSAID that has had considerable use in Europe and moderate use in the United States. Its toxicity is about average, as is its effectiveness.

Dolobid (diflunisal) is an average NSAID without particular advantages. It causes more diarrhea than is average for drugs of this class.

Meclomen (meclofenemate) is probably the most toxic NSAID, taking all complications into account. It causes serious gastrointestinal effects more frequently than most other NSAIDs and causes more frequent diarrhea than the other drugs. It is not recommended for children, and its effects have not been studied in patients with severe rheumatoid arthritis.

Tolectin (tolmetin sodium) has greater than average toxicity and seldom has benefit over alternative drugs. It needs to be taken three or four times daily since it has a fairly short half-life.

Toradol (ketorolac) is a drug used for short-term relief of pain, as in a postsurgical period. Toradol is not recommended for long-term use. It finds little use in arthritis except over periods of a week or less, and all of its side effects may not be known.

Tylenol (acetaminophen; not an NSAID)
325 mg white tablet or caplet
500 mg white tablet or caplet
500 mg yellow and red gel capsule

Purpose: To relieve pain. Acetaminophen is not a true NSAID because it does not have anti-inflammatory properties.

Indications: Mild to moderate pain, particularly with cartilage degeneration (osteoarthritis) and in RA patients on DMARDs. This is a frequently used drug.

Dosage: Not to exceed 3,000 to 4,000 mg per day.

Side effects: Acetaminophen does not directly cause serious gastrointestinal bleeding. For most people it has little toxicity. Unlike the NSAIDs, acetaminophen usually does not upset the stomach, does not cause ringing in the ears, does not affect the clotting of the blood, and does not interact with other medications. Nevertheless, nothing is perfect. Tylenol can be dangerous in overdose and *must* be stored where children cannot reach it. When taken as an intentional overdose by adults—or as an accidental overdose in children—very severe liver reactions can result. These reactions can cause liver failure, need for liver transplant, or death. Liver reaction also occurs, though very rarely, when acetaminophen is taken in common with very large amounts of alcohol. Thus, recommended doses should never be exceeded, and heavy drinkers should avoid the drug or use it in no more than half doses. It has become fashionable to suggest that persons who drink any alcohol at all should avoid acetaminophen, but this is not accurate; moderate acetaminophen doses and moderate alcohol intake can coexist safely. Moreover, use of alcohol in high amounts theoretically increases the gastrointestinal toxicity of all of the NSAIDs, so alcohol moderation is just as important for those drugs. Acetaminophen may interact adversely with Coumadin, a blood-thinning drug. Recent studies suggest that because acetaminophen is over-advertised for safety, it is taken by patients at high risk for GI bleeding, and they have severe GI side effects anyway. Like all drugs, it should be treated with respect.

Special hints: Acetaminophen is a pain reliever with approximately the same power as most of the NSAIDs—perhaps a little less. However, it has no anti-inflammatory action at all. Hence, for a long time it was thought to have a very limited role in treatment of arthritis. Recent studies have shown that for many people with osteoarthritis, Tylenol can be as effective as NSAIDs. In rheumatoid arthritis, Tylenol can be used to give pain relief while the major disease-modifying drugs (DMARDs), discussed below, are relied upon for the required anti-inflammatory activity. Tylenol is not a perfect pain reliever for everyone, but it is a drug that should be more frequently used by those for whom it is effective at relieving pain. It is relatively inexpensive.

Soon-to-be-Released Nonsteroidal Medications

Some new NSAIDs, similar to those just discussed, are in the process of review by the Food and Drug Administration. Many of these drugs are currently being used in other countries and appear to have a role in the treatment of arthritis. *Judging from current knowledge, none of these new NSAIDs will be dramatically different from drugs already available.* Also, a new drug is less well understood in terms of toxicity and benefits than a drug that has already been widely used. Some of these new drugs are likely to increase heart attack risk; we recommend not using such drugs for five years unless you are at very low heart attack risk.

Some of these drugs have been formulated to have less gastrointestinal toxicity than their predecessors, and they may be safer. Sometimes, however, the agents that cause the fewest side effects turn out to be the least powerful drugs for the management of arthritis.

In general, when considering one of the new agents, rely on your doctor's advice. If you have been having a lot of trouble with stomach upset from drugs, then it might be a good idea to try one of the agents that causes less gastrointestinal difficulty, such as Disalcid, Trilisate, Relafen, Celebrex, or Mobic. If you have not been getting the desired effect from the drugs of one chemical class, sometimes it is useful to try the drugs of a different class. But treat each of these drugs with respect and consider that it is always possible for a drug, particularly a new drug, to be responsible for a new symptom that develops while you are taking the medication.

Corticosteroids

Over 50 years ago, a "miracle" occurred: the introduction of cortisone for the treatment of rheumatoid arthritis. For people with rheumatoid arthritis and other forms of synovitis, the swelling and pain in their joints suddenly and dramatically decreased, as did the overall severity of their disease. They felt fine. The Nobel prize for medicine was awarded to the doctors who developed this drug.

This initial enthusiasm for cortisone in arthritis was tremendous. But, over the following years, the bad side effects of cortisone-like drugs were recognized. For many individuals, the side effects were clearly greater than any benefits obtained. Cortisone became the model of a drug that provides early benefits but late penalties. Now, with a half century of experience with corticosteroids (also called corticoids or steroids), our perspective is more complete. They represent a major treatment for arthritis, but their use is appropriate in only a few cases, and then only with attention to potential complications. They appear effective in treating rheumatoid arthritis over a year or so, but over the long term they actually increase disability, mortality, and susceptibility to NSAID gastrointestinal side effects.

Steroids are natural hormones manufactured by the adrenal glands. When used medically, they are given in doses somewhat higher than the amounts the body generally makes. In these doses they suppress the function of your own adrenal glands and lead to a kind of drug dependency as the adrenal gland slowly shrinks from disuse. After many months of steroid use, the drug must be withdrawn slowly to allow your own adrenal gland to return to full function; otherwise an "adrenal crisis" can occur in which you just don't have enough hormone. Steroids must be taken exactly as directed, and a physician's close advice is always required.

Steroids used in treating arthritis are very different from the sex steroids, or androgens, taken by athletes and bodybuilders, often illegally. These other steroids have no role in treating arthritis and, indeed, shouldn't be used by athletes either.

The side effects of corticosteroids can be divided into categories based on the length of time you have been taking the steroid and the dose prescribed. If you have been taking steroids for less than one week, side effects are quite rare, even if the dose has been high.

If you have been taking high doses for one week to one month, you are at risk for development of ulcers, mental changes including psychosis or depression, infection with bacterial germs, or acne. The side effects of steroid treatment become most apparent after one month to one year of medium to high dosage. The individual becomes fat in the central parts of the body, with a buffalo hump on the lower neck and wasting of the muscles in the arms and legs. Hair growth increases over the face, skin bruises appear, and stretch marks develop over the abdomen. After years of steroid treatment (even with low doses) there is loss of calcium, resulting in fragile bones. Fractures can occur with only slight injury, particularly in the spine. Cataracts slowly develop and the skin becomes thin and translucent. Some physicians believe that hardening of the arteries occurs more rapidly and that there may be complications of inflammation of the arteries. Blood pressure may increase.

Many of these side effects will occur in everyone who takes sufficient doses of cortisone or its relatives for a sufficient period. The art of managing arthritis with corticosteroids involves knowing how to minimize these side effects. Your physician will work with you to keep the dose as low as possible at all times. If possible, you may be instructed to take the drug only once daily rather than several times daily, since there are fewer side effects when it is taken this way. If you are able to take the drug only every other day, this is even better, for the side effects are then quite minimal. Unfortunately, many people find that the dosage schedules that cause the fewest side effects also give them the least relief.

Steroids are always to be used with great respect and caution. High-dose cortisone treatment for uncomplicated rheumatoid arthritis has long been considered bad medical practice in the United States; it remains the essence of some quack treatments of arthritis, such as those available in Mexican border towns. Corticosteroids are harmful in infectious arthritis and should not be given by mouth in local conditions or in osteoarthritis.

There are three ways to give corticosteroids: by mouth, by vein, or by injection into the painful area. Prednisone is the steroid usually given by mouth and is the steroid discussed here. There are perhaps ten different steroid drugs now available. Prednisone, methylprednisolone, Decadron, and Aristocort are among the most commonly used. The fluorinated steroids, such as triamcinolone, cause greater problems with muscle wasting than does prednisone. The steroids sold by brand name are about 20 times as expensive as prednisone and do not have any major advantages. Hence, there is little reason to use any of these other compounds.

Prednisone
Dosages of 1 mg, 5 mg, 10 mg, 20 mg, and 50 mg are available.

Purpose: To reduce inflammation; to suppress immunological responses.

Indications: For suppression of serious systemic manifestations of connective-tissue disease, such as kidney involvement. In selected cases, low-dose use to suppress the inflammation of rheumatoid arthritis.

Dosage: The body normally makes the equivalent of about 5 to 7.5 mg of prednisone each day. "Low-dose" prednisone treatment is from 5 to 10 mg. A "moderate dose" ranges from 15 to 30 mg per day, and a "high dose" from 40 to 60 mg per day, or even higher. The drug is often most effective when given in several doses throughout the day, but side effects are least when the same total daily dose is given as infrequently as possible.

Side effects: Prednisone causes all of the corticosteroid side effects described previously. Allergy is extremely rare. Side effects are related to dose and to duration of treatment. They can be major and can include fatal complications. Psychological dependency often occurs and complicates efforts to get off the drug.

Special hints: Before beginning treatment, discuss the need for prednisone carefully with your doctor. The decision to start steroid treatment for a chronic disease is a major one, and you want to be sure that the drug is essential. You may want a second opinion if the explanation does not completely satisfy you. When you take prednisone, follow your doctor's instructions closely. With some drugs it does not make much difference if you start and stop them on your own, but prednisone must be taken extremely regularly and exactly as prescribed. You will want to help your doctor decrease your dose of prednisone whenever possible, even if this does cause some increase in your symptoms.

When you reduce the dose of prednisone a syndrome called *steroid fibrositis* can cause increased stiffness and pain for a week to ten days after each dose reduction. Sometimes this is wrongly interpreted as a return of the arthritis, and the reduction in dosage is unnecessarily stopped. If you are going to take prednisone for a long time, ask your doctor about taking some vitamin D along with it. There is some evidence that the loss of bone, the most critical long-term side effect, can be reduced if you take vitamin D (usually prescribed as 50,000 units once or twice a month) together with adequate calcium.

If you are having some side effects, ask your doctor about once-a-day or every-other-day use of the prednisone. Watch your salt and sodium intake and keep it low, since there is already a tendency to retain fluid with prednisone. Watch your diet as well, since you will be fighting a tendency to put on fat. If you stay active and limit the calories you take in, you can minimize many of the ugly side effects of the steroid medication and can improve the strength of the bones and the muscles. If you are taking a corticosteroid other than prednisone by mouth, ask your physician if it is all right to switch to the equivalent dose of prednisone.

Steroid Injections: Depo-medrol, other brands

Purpose: To reduce inflammation in a local area.

Indications: Noninfectious inflammation and pain in a particular region of the body. Or a widespread arthritis with one or two areas causing most of the problem.

Dosage: Dosage varies depending on the preparation and purpose. The frequency of injection is more important. Usually injections should be no more than every six weeks. Many physicians set a limit of three injections in a single area.

Side effects: Steroid injections resemble a very short course of prednisone by mouth and therefore have few side effects. They result in a high concentration of the steroid in the area that is inflamed and can have quite a pronounced effect in reducing this inflammation. If a single area is injected many times, the injection appears to cause damage in that area. This has resulted in serious problems in frequently injected areas, such as the elbows of baseball pitchers. Some studies suggest that as few as ten injections in the same place can cause increased bone destruction. Hence, most doctors stop injecting well before this time.

Special hints: If one area of your body is giving you a lot of trouble, an injection sometimes makes sense. The response to the first injection will tell you quite accurately how much sense it makes. If you get excellent relief that lasts for many months, reinjection is indicated if the problem returns. The steroid injections contain a long-acting steroid, but it is in the body for only a few days. The effects may last much longer than this, however, since a cycle of inflammation and injury may be broken by the injection. If you get relief for only a few days, then injection is not going to be a very useful treatment for you. If you get no relief at all or an increase in pain, this is an obvious sign that other kinds of treatment should be sought. If you can find a "trigger point" on your body where pressure reproduces your major pain, then injection of this trigger point is sometimes beneficial. Occasionally people with osteoarthritis get benefit from injections, but injections usually are not helpful unless there is inflammation in the area.

Chapter 19

Disease-modifying Antirheumatic Drugs (DMARDs)

The anti-inflammatory drugs of Chapter 18 are symptomatic medications only. They don't do anything basic to control arthritis over the long term. For rheumatoid arthritis and other forms of synovitis, there is a much more important class of drugs. These drugs are usually called "disease-modifying antirheumatic drugs," or DMARDs. While they rarely induce true remission, in which the disease does not come back after the drug is stopped, they are much more effective anti-inflammatory agents than nonsteroidal anti-inflammatory drugs (NSAIDs). Most DMARDs have been conclusively shown to slow joint destruction in rheumatoid arthritis. DMARDs are the most important drugs for rheumatoid arthritis and are often used in other inflammatory conditions.

If you have rheumatoid arthritis or another inflammatory arthritis, you need DMARD treatments. It used to be thought that DMARDs should be reserved for late use in patients with exceptionally severe disease of many years that could not be controlled with lesser agents. Now it is recognized that these drugs should be started early and regarded as the backbone of treatment for rheumatoid arthritis. Patients with significant rheumatoid arthritis should be on one or another of these agents throughout the entire course of the disease. If you suspect rheumatoid arthritis, you should see a rheumatologist familiar with the use of DMARDs *as early as possible*.

This shift to considering DMARDs as the front-line treatment came about because of a recognition of the serious complications of rheumatoid arthritis, the substantial side effects from the NSAIDs, a reassuring safety profile for these stronger drugs, and the availability of a larger number of drugs of this class. In general, these drugs are about as safe as the moderate toxicity NSAIDs. Usually the good effects from these agents last only a few years, and so a strategy of using them sequentially, or even in combination, is required.

There are now about fifteen of these agents available, and more are under development. Methotrexate has become the most frequently used of these agents. Minocycline, also discussed below, may also be a DMARD, but this is not yet established. The cytokine treatments, despite their cost, are seeing increased use.

Gold (Intramuscular or Oral) and Penicillamine

These drugs are now used less frequently than the newer drugs. They provide dramatic benefits to over two-thirds of persons with severe rheumatoid arthritis. Each has major side effects that require stopping treatment in at least one-quarter of users and that may, in rare cases, be fatal. Gold salts and penicillamine are two very different kinds of drugs, but there are similarities in the types and magnitude of good effects and in the types of side effects. Neither appears to be of use in any disease other than rheumatoid arthritis, but the scientific proof of their effectiveness in rheumatoid arthritis is impressive.

These agents can result in complete remission of the arthritis, at least for the period while the drug is continued. In perhaps one-quarter of users the disease will actually be so well controlled that neither doctor nor patient can find any evidence of it. For reducing inflammation, the effects of these drugs can be more dramatic than with any other agents, except possibly methotrexate, leflunomide, or the cytokine treatments discussed below. These drugs pose certain significant hazards, but there is a good chance of major benefit. In rheumatoid arthritis, these drugs have been shown to retard destruction of the joint.

Myochrisine, Solganol (gold salts)

Purpose: To reduce inflammation and retard disease progression.

Indications: Rheumatoid arthritis and some other forms of synovitis.

Dosage: Usually, 50 mg per week by intramuscular injection for twenty weeks, then one to two injections per month thereafter. Many doctors use smaller doses for the first two injections to test for allergic reactions. "Maintenance" gold treatment refers to injections after the first twenty weeks (which result in a total of about 1,000 mg of gold).

Side effects: The gold salts accumulate very slowly in the tissues of the joints and in other parts of the body. Hence, side effects usually occur only after a considerable amount of gold has been received, although allergic reactions can occur even with the initial injection. The major side effects have to do with the skin, kidneys, and blood cells. The skin may develop a rash, usually occurring after ten or more injections, with big red spots or blotches, often itchy.

The kidney can be damaged so that protein leaks out of the body through the urine. This is called *nephrosis* or the *nephrotic syndrome* if it is severe. When it is recognized and the drug is stopped, the nephrosis usually goes away, but cases have been reported in which it did not reverse. The blood cell problems are the most dangerous. They can affect either the white blood cells or the platelets, those blood cells that control the clotting of the blood. In each case, the gold causes the bone marrow to stop making the particular blood cell. If the white cells are not made, the body becomes susceptible to serious infections. If the platelets are not made, the body is subject to serious bleeding episodes that can be fatal. These problems almost always reverse when the drug is stopped, but reversal may take a number of weeks, during which time the person is at risk for a major medical problem.

There are other side effects, such as ulcers in the mouth, a mild toxic effect on the liver, or nausea, but they usually are not as troublesome as the side effects just described. Overall, about one-quarter of users have to stop their course of treatment because of side effects. One or two percent of users experience a potentially serious side effect; other side effects don't really cause much of a problem. Most side effects occur during the initial period of twenty injections. Serious side effects during the maintenance period are less common.

Special hints: You must be patient with gold treatment. Good responses are almost never seen in the first ten weeks of treatment. Improvement begins slowly after that, and major improvement is usually evident by the end of 1,000 mg, or twenty weeks. Similarly, if the drug is stopped, it requires many months before the effect is totally lost.

To minimize the chance of serious side effects, most doctors recommend checking the urine for protein leakage, checking the white cells and the platelets, and asking the patient about skin rash before every injection.

Ridaura (auranofin)
3 mg brown and white capsule with tapered ends

Purpose: To reduce inflammation in rheumatoid arthritis and retard disease progression. (This drug is "oral gold.")

Indications: For anti-inflammatory activity in rheumatoid arthritis.

Dosage: Average dosage is 6 mg daily. Weeks to months may be required before full therapeutic effect is achieved.

Side effects: The most common side effect is dose-related diarrhea, which occurs at some time in approximately one-third of treated patients and requires discontinuation in 10 to 20% of patients. Skin rash has occurred in 4%, mild kidney problems in 1%, and problems with the platelets in 0.5% of patients.

Special hints: Ridaura is a helpful drug for a few rheumatoid arthritis patients, but it is seldom helpful unless it is the first DMARD used. It is not effective in osteoarthritis, gout, or minor rheumatic conditions. It is not nearly as strong a DMARD as intramuscular gold. If diarrhea is encountered, the dose should be reduced. As with intramuscular gold injections, patients should be monitored periodically for blood complications, skin rash, and protein loss in the urine. Follow your doctor's advice for the particular tests required. Ridaura is most useful in the first year or so of rheumatoid arthritis.

Penicillamine (cuprimine)
125 mg gray and yellow capsule
250 mg yellow capsule

Purpose: To reduce inflammation and retard disease progression.

Indications: Rheumatoid arthritis and some other forms of synovitis.

Dosage: Usually 250 mg (one 250 mg tablet, or two 125 mg tablets) per day for one month, then two tablets (500 mg) a day for one month, then three tablets (750 mg) per day for one month, and finally four tablets (1,000 mg) per day. Dosage usually is increased slowly, and may be increased even more slowly than this.

Side effects: Side effects closely parallel those noted above for gold injections. The major side effects are skin rash, protein leakage through the urine, or a decrease in production of the blood cells. Additionally, individuals may have nausea, or may notice a metallic taste in the mouth or a decreased sense of taste.

Special hints: This drug is now seldom used because better alternatives are available. Penicillamine takes a number of months to reach its full therapeutic effect and the effect persists for a long time after you stop taking the drug.

Monitoring for side effects has to be carefully performed. Usually a blood count or smear, a urinalysis to test for protein leakage, and questioning of the person about side effects are required every two weeks or even more frequently.

Antimalarial and Antibiotic Medications

Plaquenil (hydroxychloroquine)
200 mg round, white, scored tablet

Purpose: To reduce inflammation and to retard disease progression in rheumatoid arthritis; to reduce disease activity in systemic lupus erythematosus (lupus).

Indications: Rheumatoid arthritis and systemic lupus erythematosus.

Dosage: One to two tablets (200 to 400 mg) per day.

Side effects: This is one of the best tolerated of all drugs used for rheumatoid arthritis, and side effects are unusual. With a very few people, gastric upset or muscular weakness may result. Consideration needs to be given to the possibility of retinal (eye) toxicity, which is an occasional complication of antimalarial drugs. This rare complication appears to be always reversible if the patient is regularly monitored by periodic eye examinations after the first year of treatment. Some do not do eye checks until after five years of treatment.

Special hints: Plaquenil takes six weeks to begin to show an effect, and full effect can take up to twelve weeks, so plan on at least a twelve-week trial. This drug is consistently useful but not too powerful. Bright sunlight seems to increase the frequency of eye damage, so we recommend using sunglasses and wide-brimmed hats for sun protection. Do not exceed two tablets daily. Since the drug is so well tolerated, both tablets may be taken together in the morning. The good effects of this drug continue for weeks or months after the drug is stopped. Overall, this is one of the safest and best drugs available for treatment of rheumatoid arthritis and lupus; it should be used with respect but not fear.

Azulfidine (sulphasalazine)
Azulfidine EN-tabs: 500 mg orange, film-coated tablet

Purpose: To reduce inflammation and to retard disease progression in rheumatoid arthritis.

Indications: Rheumatoid arthritis and some other forms of synovitis.

Dosage: Three or four 500 mg tablets daily, taken in two or three doses. Dosage may be increased to as many as six 500 mg tablets, usually taken as two tablets three times daily.

Side effects: This is a sulfa drug and should not be taken by people with an allergy to sulfa, which is present in many antibiotics such as Septra and Gantrisin. Allergy is unusual, but it may take the form of a rash, wheezing, itching, fever, or jaundice. Azulfidine may cause gastric distress or other side effects in some patients. Blood tests should be done every so often to detect any effects on the blood cells or platelets; such effects are rare. Most people, probably four out of five, experience no trouble whatsoever.

Special hints: Azulfidine is used in patients with inflammatory problems with the bowels, where it reduces the inflammation, at least in part because of an antibiotic effect on the bacteria that live in the bowel. British scientists have documented that it has a major effect on rheumatoid arthritis, and this has been confirmed by investigators in the United States. It is very effective in some patients. It takes a month or more before the effects begin to be noticed, and full effects may take three or more months. Usually if you are not going to tolerate the drug, you will know in a week or so.

Minocin (minocycline)
100 mg capsule

Purpose: To reduce inflammation in rheumatoid arthritis.

Indications: This drug was developed primarily as an antibiotic and has been in use for a long time. In rheumatoid arthritis it has proved effective with mild to moderate disease and is a good drug to try earlier in the course of the disease. Some doctors think it works in rheumatoid arthritis through its antibiotic actions, but others point out that it has profound chemical effects on the joint tissues as well.

Dosage: 200 mg (one 100 mg capsule twice a day).

Side effects: Minocycline is generally well tolerated. Be careful with sun exposure. In some people it can cause severe sunburn reactions. As a broad spectrum antibiotic it decreases the number of bacteria in the bowel. This can lead to overgrowth of other bacteria and resulting diarrhea. All of this happens surprisingly rarely. More commonly there can be overgrowth of a fungus, causing severe itching around the anus or white patches in the throat and esophagus. This is a signal to discontinue the drug and sometimes to take medication for the fungus infection. Rarely, some nausea and allergic reactions occur. A few patients have developed a lupus-like illness.

Special hints: In rheumatoid arthritis it can take several weeks to see the benefit. This drug is theoretically considered a DMARD, but it has not been shown to delay the progression of rheumatoid arthritis. It can be used in combination with any of the other DMARDs. Because it is not a very powerful anti-inflammatory drug, it should not be used as the sole drug over a long period unless the results are quite dramatic. Usually patients with rheumatoid arthritis will have to move on from minocycline to stronger drugs. Minocycline is inexpensive. It should not be used in children because of the chance of mottling of the developing teeth.

Immunosuppressant Drugs

Immunosuppressant drugs are very important DMARD agents for the management of rheumatoid arthritis. They are prescribed in rheumatoid arthritis because they can reduce the number of inflammatory cells present around the joint. They are very powerful and useful drugs.

There are several important new drugs in this general category.

The immune response helps the body recognize and fight foreign particles and viruses. When it goes wrong, it can cause autoimmune disease. Antibodies from the immune system can attack the body's own tissues, causing disease. Immunosuppressant drugs can tone down this reaction.

Some of these drugs work by *cytotoxic* action. They kill rapidly dividing cells much like an X-ray beam. Since in some diseases the most rapidly dividing cells are the bad ones, the overall effect of the drugs is good. Others of these drugs antagonize a chemical system inside the cell, such as the purine system or the folate system. From the patient's standpoint, it doesn't really make much difference how the different drugs work.

A major short-term worry with many of these drugs is that they can destroy bone marrow cells. The bone marrow cells make red cells that carry oxygen, white cells that fight infection, and platelets that stop bleeding. Any of these blood cell types can be suppressed if you take enough immunosuppressant drugs.

Even if there seem to be enough white cells, infections can occur. These infections are often called "opportunistic," which means that they are caused by different kinds of germs than those that cause infections in healthy people. For example, patients with suppressed immune systems are often afflicted with herpes zoster (shingles) and can be prone to infections from types of fungi that are around all the time but seldom cause disease. Or a rare bacterial infection can occur. These infections can be difficult to treat and sometimes hard to diagnose.

Although there is some potential danger with these drugs, they actually may be no more dangerous than some of the drugs with which we have become more comfortable. The benefits can be enormous, and these drugs represent a major advance in treatment of rheumatoid arthritis.

Methotrexate
2.5 mg round yellow tablet

Purpose: For reduction of inflammation and to retard disease progression. This is an excellent drug.

Indications: Rheumatoid arthritis, dermatomyositis or polymyositis, psoriatic arthritis, other forms of synovitis.

Dosage: If taken orally, as is usual in rheumatoid arthritis, the dose is usually 7.5 to 25 mg per week given in two or three doses, twelve hours apart, sometimes as a single weekly dose. It must *not* be taken every day. It can be given as an injection as well, in which case doses may sometimes be as high as 40 or 50 mg per week (only when recommended by your doctor).

Side effects: These include opportunistic infections, mouth ulcers, and stomach problems. Damage to the liver, a special side effect of this drug, is particularly a problem if the drug is taken orally every day. When taken by mouth, this drug is absorbed by the intestine and passes through the liver on the way to the general circulation. As a result, doctors have discontinued this daily method of administration. Instead the drug is given intermittently, once a week, so that the liver has an opportunity to heal. Problems can still occur with the newer dose schedules, but they are much less frequent. A severe problem with the lungs is occasionally seen with methotrexate.

Methotrexate can, in rare cases, damage the liver. Enzymes can leak out of damaged liver cells, and this can be measured in the blood. Liver function tests are used to detect damage before it becomes severe. The tests include bilirubin (jaundice), serum albumin, and serum alkaline phosphatase. The most important, however, are the liver enzymes SGOT (also called AST) and SGPT (also called ALT). Usually test values should be below 40. With methotrexate therapy, enzyme levels are usually checked every eight to ten weeks, at least for the first one or two years, and then, if results are normal, perhaps less often. If they are abnormal more than half of the time, it can be a signal to reduce the dose, stop the drug, or to consider a liver biopsy to see if any damage has occurred.

Special hints: This drug is extremely effective in many cases of rheumatoid arthritis and has become the preferred drug for many patients. Because of its remarkable effectiveness it is now the most frequently used of the DMARDs. Some doctors used to recommend liver biopsy to be sure that the liver is normal before starting the drug. However, this procedure has some hazard and is not necessary as long as blood liver tests are normal before the drug is started. Since alcohol also can damage the liver, alcohol intake should be extremely moderate during methotrexate treatment. Some doctors recommend liver biopsy after a few years of treatment to make sure that no liver scarring has occurred. Current belief is that this is not necessary unless the liver blood tests are consistently abnormal. At this time there seem to be worse complications from liver biopsies (the death rate is between 1 in 1,000 and 1 in 10,000) than from methotrexate liver disease (only about forty serious events ever reported). Patients who are taking Plaquenil together with methotrexate seem to have fewer liver test abnormalities. Some doctors like to prescribe folic acid along with methotrexate; this may help to reduce side effects, but also increases the dose of methotrexate that you need.

Imuran (azathioprine), 6-MP (6-mercaptopurine)

50 mg hourglass-shaped, yellow to off-white, scored tablet

Purpose: For immunosuppression.

Indications: Severe systemic lupus erythematosus (lupus), rheumatoid arthritis, psoriatic arthritis, steroid-resistant polymyositis or dermatomyositis.

Dosage: 100 to 150 mg (two or three tablets) daily.

Side effects: Azathioprine (Imuran) and 6-mercaptopurine (6-MP) are closely related drugs with almost identical actions. Azathioprine is the more frequently used. Side effects include opportunistic infections and the possibility of cancer development after extended use. So far both effects are rare to absent in humans. Gastrointestinal (stomach) distress is occasionally noted. Hair loss is unusual, and there appears to be little effect on the sperm or the eggs. Although liver damage has been reported, the drug is usually well tolerated.

Special hints: Regular blood tests are required. Patients taking Imuran or 6-MP should never take allopurinol (Zyloprim), a drug used to treat gout, at the same time because the combination of these drugs can be fatal.

Once the patient responds to Imuran or 6-MP, it is often possible to reduce the dose. Theoretically, this decreases the risk of late side effects. Azathioprine has been shown to slow the progression of rheumatoid arthritis and is very effective in some patients. Most people seem not to have any side effects, but there is still concern about what might happen over the long run.

Arava (leflunomide)
10 or 20 mg tablet

Purpose: To reduce inflammation and to retard disease progression in rheumatoid arthritis.

Indications: For reduction of inflammation in moderate to severe rheumatoid arthritis.

Dosage: The standard dose is from 10 to 20 mg per day, usually 20 mg.

Side effects: Because this drug is relatively new, some side effects may not have been recognized, and long-term side effects are not known. The most frequent problems are skin rash, abdominal pain, diarrhea, and nausea. Occasionally there can be elevations of the liver enzymes or hair loss. Liver function tests are recommended at intervals of ten to twelve weeks, at least for the first year or two of treatment.

Special hints: Leflunomide has been proven to modify the course of rheumatoid arthritis. Its effectiveness appears to be quite similar to that of methotrexate, making it an important new alternative treatment for rheumatoid arthritis. It is chemically not related to other DMARDs. It appears that its action may be similar to that of Imuran, but it may be more predictably effective in rheumatoid arthritis. It may find a role in combination treatment with methotrexate or other DMARDs, although studies of such usage are not yet complete. It should not be taken by people with liver disease or with immune deficiency syndromes. It is not indicated for women who may become pregnant since the drug may persist for up to two years in the body. It has not been tested for safety and effectiveness in children. To minimize any risk of birth defects, men who wish to father a child should first stop taking the drug. Arava appears to work by inhibiting pyrimidine synthesis, causing rapidly multiplying cells, such as inflammatory cells, to divide more slowly. Treatment effects are generally seen in the first month and reach their peak after three to six months.

Sandimmune (cyclosporine)
25 mg capsule
100 mg capsule

Purpose: To reduce inflammation and disease progression in rheumatoid arthritis.

Indications: For reduction of inflammation in difficult, severe rheumatoid arthritis not responsive to other agents (not an approved use by the Food and Drug Administration).

Dosage: Use in rheumatoid arthritis is generally 3 to 5 mg per kilogram of body weight per day. For a 150-pound (70 kg) person, this is 200 to 350 mg per day.

Side effects: The principal adverse reactions are kidney failure, tremor, excess hair growth, and problems with the gums. In rheumatoid arthritis the major problem has been with the kidneys, and this sometimes requires discontinuation of the drug. The kidney failure is usually reversible.

Special hints: Cyclosporine was developed as a drug to prevent rejection of kidney, heart, and other organ transplants. It is a strong immunosuppressant. In rheumatoid arthritis its use is reserved for severely affected persons and it should be given only by physicians who are thoroughly familiar with its use. It can be effective in some patients. The problem for rheumatoid arthritis patients is the kidney damage, which occurs at lower doses than in transplant patients. Hence, the dose must be kept lower. Some patients have had severe disease flare-ups after stopping cyclosporine. Researchers are exploring several ways to reduce the kidney problems. Use of this drug for arthritis is decreasing.

Cellcept (mycophenolate mofetil)
250 mg blue-brown capsules
500 mg lavender caplet-shaped tablets

Purpose: To reduce inflammation and immunological reactions in organ transplant patients and, potentially, in others.

Indications: This drug has not been approved by the FDA to treat arthritis but is being used "off label" in systemic lupus erythematosus to allow steroid reduction and to replace more toxic cytotoxic drugs. It has been used occasionally in rheumatoid arthritis.

Dosage: Up to 3,000 mg/day.

Side effects: Somewhat like azathioprine (Imuran).

Special hints: This is an unproven drug that appears to work in lupus, perhaps as well as cyclophosphanide. Talk with a rheumatologist before taking it to be sure that it makes sense for you. It seems to be well tolerated and effective, but we don't know for sure. Ironically, we never will know because the drug is already available "off label" and the company is not interested in doing rigorous studies to prove new indications. This sounds bad, but remember that methotrexate, now a standard treatment, was in the same position for many years—apparently effective but unproven.

Cytokine Treatments

Cytokines are natural chemical substances that deliver important messages from cell to cell in the body. These messages often help in the regulation of chronic inflammation and tissue damage. These new drugs fight inflammation at the molecular level and represent a very major advance. For many people with rheumatoid arthritis they are the strongest drugs yet. Side effects are usually manageable. They need to be given by vein or by injection, but most people don't mind this very much.

They do pose an ethical problem—they are very expensive—and you need to decide how you feel about this. These drugs cost from $10,000 to $16,000 per year. If you do not have insurance that covers these drugs, then you may not be able to afford them or you may have to forego other things that are important to you to pay for the drugs. If you do have insurance that covers them, you have to recognize that their costs are helping to raise insurance premiums for everybody. Average medical costs in the United States are about $6,000 a year per person. If you are using more resources than this, someone else has to make do with less.

Here are our suggestions. First, a rheumatologist who is very familiar with how these drugs work should suggest one of these medications to you. Second, if you ask your rheumatologist and he or she doesn't think you would gain very much by using these drugs, wait a while and see how you do on more standard DMARD treatment. Third, if you start one of these medications, allow it no more than two or three months to give you a major benefit. If you don't get such a benefit, stop the drug. Many people actually don't do as well as they were doing on the older drugs. Our experience is that no more than 10 or 15% of patients with RA require these drugs if they have a rheumatologist who knows how to use the older drugs wisely. Some other rheumatologists, however, think that most RA patients should be treated with the new and costly treatments. Good luck.

Enbrel (etanercept)

Purpose: For control of inflammation and to retard the progression of severe rheumatoid arthritis not completely responsive to other drugs.

Indications: Moderate to severe rheumatoid arthritis.

Dosage: The standard dose is 25 mg given twice weekly by subcutaneous injection. Most patients can quickly learn to perform the injections themselves, although the first dose administration should be supervised by a health-care professional. A once weekly injection of 50 mg is also used.

Side effects: About one-third of patients develop minor injection-site reactions. Theoretically, severe infections can result, although these do not appear to be very frequent. There is some concern about possible development of lymphoma or other cancers, but to date there has been no suggestion of this. Allergic reactions, sometimes severe, can occur but appear to be very rare. In general, the drug is considered to be quite well tolerated.

Special hints: This is an extremely powerful and often dramatic drug for treatment of rheumatoid arthritis, even after other drugs have failed to completely control the disease. It appears to be effective in children with arthritis as well. It works by blocking the receptor for TNF-alpha. Some patients develop antibodies to their own tissues while taking the drug, but this is not seen today to be a major difficulty since the antibodies are present only in small amounts. A major problem is cost. A year of treatment costs approximately $12,000, making this one of the most expensive treatments for rheumatoid arthritis. Nevertheless, the often dramatic results may make this a good value for patients with very serious rheumatoid arthritis for whom other DMARDs have failed. Initial clinical studies have followed patients for up to a year with continuing good results, although long-term side effects and effectiveness have not yet been determined.

Remicade (infliximab)

Purpose: For treatment of severe rheumatoid arthritis, generally taken at the same time as methotrexate. For treatment of severe Crohn's disease of the bowel.

Indications: Severe rheumatoid arthritis not adequately controlled with other DMARD medications.

Dosage: Usual dose is 3 mg per kilogram of body weight, given by intravenous injection under medical supervision, at two-month intervals.

Side effects: Minor adverse events including headache, diarrhea, rash, and others are common but are generally well tolerated. There may be a slight increase in the rate of infections. There are theoretical concerns about development of lymphomas or other cancers, but it is not yet known if these occur, and, if they do, whether the rate is greater than those sometimes seen in patients using Imuran or methotrexate. Such lymphomas are sometimes seen in rheumatoid arthritis without any immunosuppressive or cytokine treatment whatsoever.

Special hints: This very powerful new drug is an antibody to tumor necrosis factor (TNF). It is very effective in the treatment of Crohn's disease and has dramatically changed the treatment of that chronic inflammatory condition. Almost all of the studies for treatment of rheumatoid arthritis have been in combination with methotrexate, and, when Remicade is added to methotrexate, further dramatic improvement usually occurs.

Improvement is usually seen after the first infusion but may continue after several more infusions. Antibodies to DNA have occurred and there have been a small number of cases with a reversible condition similar to lupus. It is believed that methotrexate helps promote tolerance to continued treatment with Remicade. Long-term side effects and effectiveness against rheumatoid arthritis beyond one year of treatment have not yet been established. Remicade treatment is expensive, with the cost of a year of treatment exceeding $10,000. Nevertheless, this dramatic new treatment may have substantial value for patients with severe rheumatoid arthritis not adequately controlled by other DMARDs, particularly when added to methotrexate.

Kineret (anakinra)

Purpose: For control of inflammation and to retard the progression of severe rheumatoid arthritis not completely responsive to other DMARDs.

Indications: Moderate to severe rheumatoid arthritis. May be used alone or in combination with other DMARDs except Enbrel or Remicade.

Dosage: The usual dose is 100 mg per day given by subcutaneous injection under medical supervision, generally at intervals of one to three months.

Side effects: Serious infections can occur in about 1 to 2% of patients. Decreased white cell counts can occur. Injection site reactions occur in most people but are usually mild and are uncommon after four weeks of treatment. Infections are most common when Enbrel and Kineret are used together, and this combination should be used with great caution. Allergic and other types of side effects can occur. In general it is considered to be well tolerated.

Special hints: This is a powerful new drug approved by the FDA in December 2001, although perhaps not quite as powerful as Remicade. It is a receptor antagonist for interleukin-1, a cytokine that increases inflammation, and is technically called "IL1ra." It has a distinct way of working and might be effective when other cytokine treatments are not. It works well with methotrexate and other traditional DMARDs. Like other cytokine treatments it is expensive and cannot be taken by mouth.

Humira (adalimumab)

Purpose: For reduction of inflammation, slowing of disease progression, and preservation of physical function in patients with rheumatoid arthritis (RA) and some other conditions. This drug inhibits tumor necrosis factor alpha, as do Remicade and Enbrel.

Dosage: By injection, usually self-administered, each two weeks. For reference, Enbrel requires injections once or twice a week.

Side effects: The most common and serious are infections, including tuberculosis, deep fungal infections, and a number of others. Serious bacterial infections and sepsis, including fatalities, have been reported.

Special hints: This drug costs about $16,000 per year of treatment. Before you start, get a chest X-ray and a TB skin test. Bring any possible infection to your doctor's attention promptly. Concerns about side effects with the nervous system or the development of a cancer have been raised but such side effects appear unusual. Talk with your doctor about current knowledge of side effects, as more information will become available over time.

Rituxan (rituximab)

Purpose: To fight inflammation and immunological or malignant conditions mediated by "B-cells," which are the source of all antibodies. This is an anticancer drug, developed for and effective in treatment of B-cell lymphomas, a kind of lymph node cancer.

Indications: For treatment of B-cell lymphoma. It is hoped that this drug will be useful in treatment of rheumatoid arthritis. Because it is available for "off-label" use in RA, some doctors have been trying it and think that it is quite effective.

Dosage: By intravenous infusion, as prescribed.

Side effects: Fatal infusion reactions have been reported, usually with the first infusion. Severe skin reactions have been seen, and, rarely, these have been fatal. Infections and other side effects can occur.

Special hints: This drug is not yet ready for prime time to treat RA, but it may become so. It is a promising monoclonal antibody, and it represents an entirely new approach to RA treatment. We do not recommend its use before approval by the FDA for treatment of rheumatoid arthritis. Even if approval comes, you may not want to be one of the first to try it.

abatacept (no brand name yet)

Purpose: To reduce severity and progression of rheumatoid arthritis.

Indications: Moderate to severe rheumatoid arthritis with methotrexate failure.

Dosage: Injections each two weeks; used in combination with methotrexate.

Side effects: Well tolerated in early studies, but with rare severe infections.

Special hints: This drug is not approved as of this writing (2005). It is an entirely new approach to treat rheumatoid arthritis involving fusion proteins. Early studies are quite encouraging, and the FDA may put it on the fast track for early approval. It may be the most promising and may become the first approved of new drugs currently under investigation for disease modification in rheumatoid arthritis. It will be expensive.

Chapter 20

Painkillers and Other Approaches to Reduce Pain

Pain-reducing drugs, except plain acetaminophen (Tylenol), have little place in the treatment of arthritis. Tylenol, described in Chapter 18, is an important anti-arthritis drug.

There are four major disadvantages of the strong painkillers. First, they don't do anything for the arthritis; they just cover it up. Second, they suppress the pain mechanism that tells you when you are doing something that is injuring your body. If you suppress the pain mechanism, you may injure your body without being aware of it. Third, the body adjusts to pain medicines, so that they aren't as effective over the longer term. This phenomenon is called *tolerance* and develops to some extent with all painkillers. Fourth, pain medicines can have major side effects. The side effects range from stomach distress to constipation to mental changes. Most of these drugs are "downers," which you don't need if you have arthritis. You need to be able to cope with a somewhat more difficult living situation than the average person. These drugs decrease your ability to solve problems.

Many individuals develop dependence on these agents. In arthritis, the addiction is somewhat different from what we usually imagine. Most people with arthritis are not truly physically addicted to codeine or Percodan or Demerol. Rather, they are psychologically dependent on these drugs as a crutch and become inordinately concerned with the attempt to eliminate every last symptom. These agents can conflict with efforts to maintain independent living.

By and large, use these drugs only for the short term and only when resting the sore part, so that you don't reinjure it while the pain is suppressed. Drugs mentioned first in this list are less harmful than those listed later. Drugs to reduce inflammation, discussed in Chapter 18, may reduce pain through direct pain action as well as through reduction of inflammation. In osteoarthritis, plain acetaminophen (Tylenol, other brands) is often useful as a pain reliever.

The principles in the preceding paragraphs regarding the use and misuse of pain relievers also hold for a number of less common pain relievers not described in the following section.

Drugs to Reduce Pain

Darvon (Darvon compound, Darvotran, Darvocet, Darvocet-N, propoxyphene)

Darvon: 32 mg, 65 mg pink capsule

Darvon compound: 32 mg gray and pink capsule; 65 mg gray and red capsule

Darvocet-N: 50 mg, 100 mg capsule-shaped, dark orange, coated tablet

Purpose: Pain relief.

Indications: For short-term use to decrease mild pain.

Dosage: One-half grain (32 mg) or 1 grain (65 mg) every four hours as needed for pain.

Side effects: These drugs have been widely used with a reasonably good safety record. In some cases side effects may be due to use of aspirin or other medication in combination with the Darvon. Most worrisome to us has been the mentally dull feeling that many individuals report, sometimes described as a gray, semi-unhappy fog. Others do not seem to notice this effect. Side reactions include dizziness, headache, sedation, paradoxical excitement, skin rash, and gastrointestinal disturbances.

Special hints: Darvon is not anti-inflammatory. The pain relief given is approximately equal to that of aspirin or acetaminophen in most cases. The drug is more expensive than aspirin or acetaminophen. It can induce dependence, particularly after long-term use.

Codeine (Empirin #3, 4; Tylenol #1, 2, 3, 4; aspirin with codeine #2, 3, 4; Vicodin)

Codeine (Empirin): 30 mg, 60 mg round, white tablet
Tylenol: 8 mg, 15 mg, 30 mg, 60 mg round, white tablet
Vicodin: 5 mg, 500 mg capsule-shaped, white tablet

Purpose: Moderate pain relief.

Indications: For moderate, short-term pain relief.

Dosage: The dosage of codeine is often coded by number. For example, Empirin with codeine #1 (or Empirin #1) contains one-eighth grain or 8 mg of codeine phosphate per tablet; #2 contains one-fourth grain or 16 mg; #3 contains one-half grain or 32 mg; and #4 contains 1 grain or 65 mg of codeine. A common dosage is a #3 tablet (32 mg codeine) every four hours as needed for pain.

Side effects: The side effects are proportional to the dosage. The more you take, the more side effects you are likely to have. Allergic reactions are quite rare.

Codeine is a mild narcotic. Thus, it can lead to addiction, with tolerance and drug dependence. Frequently in older persons with arthritis it leads to constipation and sometimes a set of complications including fecal impaction and diverticulitis. More worrisome is the way that persons using codeine seem to lose their will to cope. The person taking codeine for many years sometimes seems sluggish and generally depressed. We don't really know whether the codeine is responsible, but we do think that codeine often makes it more difficult for the person with arthritis to cope with the very real problems that abound.

Percodan (Percobarb, Percodan-Demi, Percogesic)

Percodan: Yellow tablet
Percodan-Demi: Pink tablet

Purpose: For pain relief.

Indications: For short-term relief of moderate to severe pain.

Dosage: One tablet every six hours as needed.

Side effects: Percodan is a curious combination drug. The basic narcotic is oxycodone, to which is added aspirin and other minor pain relievers. Combination drugs have a number of theoretical disadvantages, but Percodan is a strong and effective pain reliever. It does require a special prescription because it is a strong narcotic and the hazards of serious addiction are present. The manufacturers state that the habit-forming potential is somewhat less than with morphine and somewhat greater than with codeine. The drug is usually well tolerated. Percoset is a similar drug with acetaminophen instead of aspirin.

Special hints: Percodan is a good drug for people with cancer, but it can be dangerous in the treatment of arthritis. It is not an anti-inflammatory agent and does not work directly on any of the disease processes. It is habit-forming and it does break the pain reflex. It is a mental depressant and can result in serious addiction.

Demerol (meperidine)
Demerol-Hydrochloride: 50 mg, 100 mg round, white, scored tablet
Demerol APAP: 50 mg tablet, pink with dark pink splotches

Purpose: For relief of severe pain such as in cancer, heart attacks, kidney stones.

Indications: For temporary relief of severe pain, as with a bad fracture that has been immobilized.

Dosage: Various preparations are available that contain 25 mg, 50 mg, or 100 mg of Demerol. One tablet every four hours for pain is a typical dose. Dose is increased for more severe pain and decreased for milder pain.

Side effects: Demerol is a major narcotic approximately equivalent to morphine in pain relief capacity and in addiction potential. Tolerance develops and increasing doses may be required. Drug dependence and severe withdrawal symptoms may be seen if the drug is stopped. Psychological dependence also occurs. The underlying disease may be covered up and serious symptoms may be masked. Nausea, vomiting, constipation, and a variety of other side effects may occur.

Special hints: This is not a drug for the treatment of arthritis. Stay away from it.

Tranquilizers

Valium, Librium, and other tranquilizers are among the most prescribed drugs in North America. They do not help arthritis. These drugs depress the patient and should be avoided by people with arthritis whenever possible.

Muscle Relaxants

Soma, Flexeril, and a number of other agents are prescribed frequently as "muscle relaxants." In general these act like tranquilizers. They treat only symptoms and are usually not helpful in arthritis. One exception: Flexeril is sometimes useful against fibromyalgia.

Antidepressants

There is a role for antidepressant treatment in arthritis when depression is a problem, and in selected cases it can be very helpful. Sometimes a low dose of an antidepressant, such as Elavil, is given at bedtime, not to fight depression but to help improve the quality of sleep and to reduce the problems of fibromyalgia.

Hyaluronic Acid Injections (Viscosupplementation)

Hyalgan (Hyaluronan); Synvisc (Hylan G-F 20)
These two substances have recently received FDA approval for treatment of pain associated with osteoarthritis of the knee in patients who have not responded to traditional therapy. The drugs are given by injection directly into the knee joint and are intended to improve the viscosity of the synovial fluid so that lubrication in the joint is better. The injections are not inexpensive and have been shown in some studies to be about as effective as NSAIDs, that is, a minor response. Most studies have shown no benefit at all. They may possibly have a role in osteoarthritis of the knee, particularly if only one knee is more severely involved. They are sometimes used as a last resort before total knee replacement surgery. Relief may extend for only a few days or may appear to last for

many months, although the drug itself is present in the joint only for a few days. Medicare and many insurance companies recently have agreed to cover the initial use of these compounds.

Alternative Medicines

Glucosamine, chondroitin sulphate

Many folk remedies are used for treatment of arthritis, and some individuals appear to benefit from some of them. Hence, it is difficult to be critical of the use of unproven or relatively unproven agents unless they are hazardous or are used in such a way as to displace the use of more effective medical treatments. In this latter case, they can be a cruel delusion.

The recent boom in the use of glucosamine and chondroitin sulphate is best considered an alternative medicine phenomenon. These agents are widely available over the counter, from supermarkets to health food stores. They are normal constituents of the joint cartilage and are sold as dietary supplements. There do not appear to be any major side effects. They have been used most frequently in osteoarthrosis but also have been used in a number of musculoskeletal pain syndromes.

The scientific base for the effectiveness of these compounds is currently very weak. Some quite old studies in the European medical literature suggested that they might be effective in the treatment of osteoarthritis, but most recent studies have been less impressive. It has been pointed out that there is no way these drugs could get from the stomach to the joint since they have to be broken down in the intestine into smaller molecules before they can be absorbed into the body. Hence, it is not possible for them to work by the mechanism suggested for their action. High-quality clinical studies are currently under way; results are not yet definitive but some studies suggest a positive but weak effect in some patients.

Many patients who take these drugs alone or together do not tell their doctor that they are taking them, largely because they fear the disapproval of the doctor. If you do take these agents, please tell your doctor, so that we can begin to build a critical medical appreciation of their effectiveness or lack of it. If any medication, whether traditional or alternative in character, appears to be giving major benefits, then it usually makes sense to continue the medication as long as benefit appears to continue. We hope to have information about the true effectiveness of these agents in the relatively near future. For now, most arthritis doctors take the position "don't encourage, don't discourage."

Names and Availability

Some drugs are known by different names in the United States, Canada, the United Kingdom, New Zealand, Australia, and in non-English-speaking countries. In addition, because of drugs' differing status in terms of government approval, some drugs available in one country are not available in another. For information about any drug whose name does not appear in this chapter, speak to your doctor or pharmacist.

Chapter 21

What About Surgery?

Surgery can relieve pain, restore function, and return a patient to employment. Its potential to satisfactorily repair a damaged joint increases year by year. But surgery is expensive and painful, is associated with a long recovery period, keeps you away from activities during the period of convalescence, and may not be successful. The joint might be worse afterward. Surgery can even kill you or paralyze you, although this is rare. The decision to undergo surgery is one that you will make with your doctor. It's a major step, and you want to make the right decision. Here are some guidelines to help you sort out the issues.

General Rules

Surgery for Arthritis Is Seldom Urgent

With only a few exceptions, a delay of days, weeks, or even months makes relatively little difference with surgery for arthritis. If the operation is successful, you will still have the good results to enjoy; if the operation is unsuccessful, you will have delayed the pain and expense by waiting. You have plenty of time for a second opinion or a third. You can watch your condition to see if it goes away by itself or perhaps stabilizes at an acceptable level. So take your time. Rare exceptions to this rule include bone conditions causing nerve pressure, a bacterial infection in the bone or joint, or a rupture of the tendons.

Not All Surgeons Are Equal

Generally, you will want an orthopedic or hand surgeon to perform any operations on your joints that may be required. You will also want a surgeon who does a lot of joint operations and is up-to-date on the latest techniques. Surgery is a rapidly changing field, and familiarity with the most recent advances leads to better results. A surgeon who performs the operation only once or twice a year is not likely to have the same level of skill as a surgeon who does the operation weekly. As a dividend, you will usually find that the busy joint surgeon is more conservative in his or her recommendation for an operation. It's not at all uncommon for a good orthopedic surgeon to state candidly that the condition for which the operation is being considered is not likely to respond to surgical treatment—and then you will be spared an unsuccessful operation.

Not All Operations Are Equal

Total hip replacement and total knee replacement are very fine operations; almost all patients receive benefit from them. On the other hand, certain procedures, such as tendon operations on the small joints of the hand or most kinds of back surgery are far less predictable. Before you decide to have either of the latter two kinds of operation, you will want to find out how good the recommended operation is.

Best Results Are Achieved When Problems Are Localized

Treatment with medications is often best for a widespread problem. On the other hand, if the problem is localized, say in one knee, then surgery is likely to be a good, targeted approach to the problem. If a large number of joints are involved, surgery may be impractical. For example, the lower extremity has eight major weight-bearing areas: the two forefeet, the ankles, the knees, and the hips. If any one of these areas is limiting walking, surgery may be a wise move. But if all eight areas are bad, then fixing one joint without providing relief to the other seven will not translate into function and increased activity. Be realistic. Ask how much better off you would be if the area of a proposed operation were entirely well. If the answer is, "Not much," then surgery may not be advisable.

Best Surgical Results Are Achieved in Treatment of Large Joints

Joints are complicated structures and scarring after surgery can result in stiffness, particularly if the surface area of the joint is small. The best surgical procedures repair large joints, such as the hip and the knee. Results in these areas are usually predictably good. With the smaller joints, sophisticated repair techniques sometimes don't improve function significantly and should be approached with caution. Usually problems with smaller joints are also problems that involve many joints, which again complicates the surgical approach.

Specific Operations

Joint Replacement

This is the most important orthopedic surgical procedure for arthritis. The joint is removed and replaced entirely by an artificial joint. The cartilage is replaced by long-wearing plastics such as Teflon, the bone is replaced by stainless steel, and the artificial joint is embedded in the ends of the bones on either side by a marvelous cement called methyl methacralate. This bone cement made the new era in joint surgery possible by providing a way to anchor the artificial joint to the bones.

The hip was the first joint to be replaced. Total hip replacement is an excellent operation in the hands of an experienced surgeon. Pain is almost totally relieved, and function is greatly improved. The present artificial hip is estimated to last ten to fifteen years, and newer models are expected to last longer as design problems are overcome. The failure rate is only 1 or 2%, but these patients may have infections or even have to have the artificial hip removed. It is true that some patients receiving artificial hips have to have a replacement for the replacement; it is also true that the final result usually has been satisfactory. Recently a new type of total hip operation has been developed that works by allowing bony ingrowth into the artificial joint and that does not require cement.

The knee is a complicated hinge joint with a requirement for sideways stability. This has made it more difficult to construct an appropriate replacement joint, since the joint must move freely in the hinge direction but must strongly resist sideways force. The ball-and-socket joint of the hip poses easier engineering problems. Techniques of knee replacement have been greatly refined over the last several years.

Ankle replacements remain less frequently used. Shoulder replacements have become quite good. Operations to replace the small joints of the fingers are widely practiced, but the outcome has not been uniformly satisfactory. One of the problems with present operations for the small joints of the hands is that appearance may be considerably improved by the straightening of deformed fingers, but the ability to use the hand may not be greatly changed.

Synovectomy

Removal of inflamed synovium is termed a synovectomy. This operation results in a reduction of the swelling of synovitis and presumably less enzymatic damage to the joint because the inflamed tissue mass has been reduced. Unfortunately, joint stiffness is often experienced after the synovectomy and the inflamed tissue frequently grows back. There has been a long-standing argument about whether synovectomy should be done early or late (or never) in rheumatoid arthritis, with some doctors holding each extreme position. In other words, the effects of synovectomy are not so dramatic that people can't argue about them. There should be a special reason for this operation, such as worsening of a single joint when all other joints are in control. Use of this operation has decreased as medical treatments have improved.

Resections

Some older operations sound a bit strange, and this is the case with resection procedures. Here, bones are just cut away and removed. This sounds as though it wouldn't be very helpful, but it often is. Resection of the metatarsal heads in the forefoot, for example, can relieve pain and restore the ability to walk. Similar operations may be done in the distal ulna, the bone on the outside of the wrist. Bunions and other protuberances can be removed. While this type of surgery is not elegant in concept, it can be useful in some instances.

Fusions

An operation to unite two bones is termed a *fusion*. Such operations are useful to stabilize joints; the fusion provides a platform for movement and prevents pain in the fused area. The wrist and ankle are the joints where this procedure is most frequently used; fusion of the back or part of the neck is also performed on occasion. A successful fusion, limiting all motion, stops pain. But in the area that is fused, flexibility is lost. Usually a fusion places additional strain on nearby joints that are called on to take over the flexibility functions. Fusion doesn't always work, and nonunion can occur. These operations are useful, however, in certain situations.

Back Surgery

A full discussion about indications for back surgery is beyond the scope of this chapter. Most patients know from talking with friends that unsuccessful back surgery is common. In most cases the doctor was not very enthusiastic about performing this surgery, but the continuing problems of the patient eventually led doctor and patient to agree on this measure. And it didn't work.

By and large, back surgery is not advisable unless there is evidence of pressure on nerve roots. This may happen with a herniated disk, or with narrowing of the spinal canal, or with back fractures.

Myelography is a special X-ray technique for obtaining an X-ray image of the spinal cord. A myelogram can demonstrate pressure on the nerves in the spinal cord. Operations in patients with negative myelograms are the least likely to succeed. However, the myelogram itself requires placement of a needle into the spinal canal and the injection of a not-innocuous dye into the space around the spinal cord. It is uncomfortable, and there are some side effects. Hence, even considering a myelogram should be reserved for the most serious back problems. A computed tomography (CT) scan or magnetic resonance (MR) imaging test can provide much of the same information. The CT scan involves some radiation and is expensive, but generally safe. It does not hurt. MR imaging tests don't involve radiation. They are expensive but can be very helpful; the view of the back structures is extraordinarily clear.

The back is composed of an extraordinarily complex set of muscles, ligaments, and tendons. Back injury may be anywhere and is frequently not in the spine; hence, surgery on the spine may not be countering what is wrong. Seek multiple opinions before having a back operation. You want to avoid back surgery if you can, and it's mainly up to you.

Neurological Operations

There can be pressure on nerves out in the limbs. An example is the carpal tunnel syndrome, where there is pressure on the nerve passing over the front of the wrist resulting in pain and tingling in the fingers. This pressure can be effectively eliminated by surgery, and surgery should be considered if rest or injection do not result in disappearance of the syndrome within a few weeks. Other problems, such as a Morton's neuroma, can also cause peripheral pain. Here, an injury has caused the nerve fibers to grow into a little ball and to transmit pain signals all the time. If this bundle of nerves is removed, the pain is eliminated and a good result obtained. So while we can't really operate to repair nerves, we can either remove the structures that are pressing on them or remove the area that is sending the abnormal signals.

"Cosmetic" Surgery

Usually surgery for a joint should be done only to relieve pain or to improve function. The appearance of the joint is much less important. Some operations serve mainly to improve appearance. Many patients are later disappointed by such operations. The appearance is less than perfect anyway, and the patient somehow has been expecting that the part would work better if it looked better, despite advice to the contrary.

Chapter 22

Making Treatment Decisions

We hear about new treatments, new drugs, nutritional supplements, and alternative treatments all the time. Hardly a week goes by without a new treatment of some kind being reported in the news. Drug companies and nutritional supplement companies run television commercials and place large ads in newspapers and magazines. Our email boxes are filled with promises of new treatments or cures from spammers. We are bombarded in the market or pharmacy with signs and packaging for over-the-counter alternative treatments.

What can we believe? How can we decide what might be worth a try?

An important part of managing our own care is being able to evaluate these claims so that we can make an informed decision about trying something new. There are some important questions that should be asked in the process of making a decision about any treatment, mainstream medical as well as complementary and alternative treatments.

1. Where did you learn about this?

Was it reported in a scientific journal, supermarket tabloid, an ad in print or on TV, or a flyer you picked up somewhere? Did your doctor suggest it? The source of the information is important. Results that are reported in a respected scientific journal are more likely to be believable that those you might see in the supermarket tabloid or on an advertising flyer. Results reported in scientific journals, such as the *New England Journal of Medicine, Lancet,* or *Science* are usually from research studies. These studies are carefully reviewed for scientific integrity by other scientists, who are very careful about what they approve for publication. Many alternative treatments and nutritional supplements, however, have not been studied scientifically, so they are not as well represented in the scientific literature as medical treatments are. If this is the case, you need to be extra careful and critical about analyzing what you read.

2. Were the people who got better like you?

In the past, many studies were done with easy-to-get people, so older studies were often done on college students, nurses, or white men. This has changed, but it is still important to find out if the people that got better were like you. Were they from the same age group? Did they have a similar lifestyle? Did they have the same health problems as you do? Were they the same sex and race? If the people aren't like you, the results may not be the same for you.

3. Could anything else have caused these positive changes?

We talked to a woman who had jut returned from a two-week stay at a spa in the tropics and reported that her arthritis improved dramatically because of the special diet and supplements she had received. But it's hard to attribute her improvement totally to the treatment, when the warm weather, relaxation, and pampering may have had a lot to do with her improvement! It is important to look at everything that has changed since starting the treatment. It is common to take up a generally healthier lifestyle when starting a new treatment—could that be playing a part in the improvement? Have you started another medication or treatment at the same time? Has the weather improved? Are you under less stress than before you started the treatment? Can you think of anything else that could have affected your health?

4. Does treatment suggest stopping other medications or treatments?

Does it require that you stop taking another basic medication because of dangerous interactions? If the other medication is important, this will require a discussion with your health care provider before making a change.

5. Does treatment result in not eating a well-balanced diet?

Does it eliminate any important nutrients or stress only a few nutrients that could be harmful to you? Maintaining a balanced diet is important for your overall health. Make sure that you're not sacrificing important vitamins or make sure that you're getting them from another source if you change your eating habits. Also make sure that you're not putting excessive stress on your organs by concentrating on only a few nutrients.

6. Can I think of any possible dangers or harm?

Some treatments take a toll on your body. All treatments have side effects and possible risks. Make sure that you and your health care provider have a thorough discussion about what these may be. Only you can decide if the potential problems are worth the possible benefit, but you must have all that information in order to make that decision. Many people think that if something is natural, it must be good for you. This may not be true. "Natural" isn't necessarily better just because it comes from a plant or animal. Tobacco is natural. In the case of the powerful heart medication, digitalis, which comes from the foxglove plant, it is "natural" but the dosage must be exact or it could be dangerous. Hemlock comes from a plant, but it is a deadly poison. Some may be safe in small doses, but dangerous in larger doses. Be careful.

There is no regulatory agency that is responsible for determining if what is listed on the label of a nutritional supplement is actually what's in the bottle, except in Germany. Supplements don't have the same safeguards as for medications. Do some research about the company selling the product before you try it.

7. Can I afford it?

Do you have the money to give this treatment the time it needs to see an improvement? Is your health strong enough to maintain this new regimen? Will you be able to handle it emotionally? Will this put a strain on your relationships at home and at work?

8. Am I willing to go to trouble and expense?

Do you have the necessary support in place?

If you ask yourself all of these questions and decide to try a new treatment, remember it is very important to inform your health care professional about it if this is something you are doing on your own. Remember that you are partners, and you will need to keep him or her informed on your progress during the time you are taking the treatment.

The internet can respond to new treatments very quickly and is therefore a place to go for up-to-date information about these treatments. If you use the internet as a source of information about medications or other treatments, it is important to be cautious. Not everything found on the internet is correct or even safe. Therefore, to help you find the more reliable sources look at the author or sponsor of the site and the URL address. Addresses ending in .edu, .org, and .gov are generally more objective and reliable; they originate from universities, nonprofit organizations, and governmental agencies. Some .com sites can also be good, but because they come from commercial or for-profit organizations, their information might be biased, as they may be trying to promote or sell their own products. One good source for information about questionable treatments is Quackwatch.org, a nonprofit corporation whose purpose is to combat health-related frauds, myths, fads, and fallacies (www.quackwatch.org). They also have other sites that are accessible from Quackwatch. For more information on finding resources on the internet and elsewhere, see Chapter 8.

Index